The Healer's Verses: Medical Mysteries in Rhyme for the Analytical Mind

Riddle Me This: A Professional Exploration in Poetry, Volume 2

Said Al Azri

Published by Said Al Azri, 2024.

While every precaution has been taken in the preparation of this book, the publisher assumes no responsibility for errors or omissions, or for damages resulting from the use of the information contained herein.

THE HEALER'S VERSES: MEDICAL MYSTERIES IN RHYME FOR THE ANALYTICAL MIND

First edition. February 5, 2024.

ISBN: 979-8223723240

Written by Said Al Azri.

Also by Said Al Azri

Classics Reimagined: A Comedic Twist
Echoes of Venice: A Modern Tale of Redemption
Moby-Dick Reversed: A Whale's Humorous Account
Treasure Island: The Parrot's Perspective
Tom Sawyer: The Great Exaggerator

Family and Parenting Dynamics
From My Heart to Yours: Messages of Love and Learning for My Child
Balancing Family Life: Strategies for Modern Parenting

Heartstrings: Tales of Valentine's Verse
Verses of the Heart: A Poetic Journey Through Love's Whimsy
Verses of the Heart 2: A Poetic Journey Through Love's Whimsy

Life, Hobbies, and Careers Series
From Amateur to Applause: A Beginner's Guide to Stand-Up Comedy

Table of Contents

To my beloved wife, Maida, and our cherished children,

This book is a testament to the enduring strength and compassion that you embody, which inspires me daily.

May the dedication and care reflected in these pages serve as a mirror to the love and support you have always provided me.

Here's to the journey of exploration and discovery we continue to share together.

With all my love and gratitude, Said

Introduction

Welcome to the captivating realm of "The Healer's Verses: Medical Mysteries in Rhyme for the Analytical Mind," where the intricate world of medicine and the artistry of poetry blend in a symphony of verse and insight. This book is not merely a collection of poems; it's an odyssey through the vast and complex landscape of healthcare, re-envisioned through the lens of rhythmic beauty.

In an era where health and science stand at the forefront of our collective consciousness, influencing every facet of our lives—from the battles fought in the silent corridors of hospitals to the quiet resilience in recovery rooms—medicine has also emerged as a muse for creativity and poetic expression. "The Healer's Verses" is a homage to this confluence, offering a unique exploration of medical phenomena and terminologies through the elegance and simplicity of poetry.

In "The Healer's Verses: Medical Mysteries in Rhyme for the Analytical Mind," you will discover a collection of 252 riddle poems, each intricately woven around a medical term or concept. This book stands as a treasury of poetic puzzles, as well as a distinctive instrument for sharpening your medical acumen and analytical prowess. Each riddle poem within these pages poses a delightful yet thought-provoking challenge, inviting you to decipher the enigmas of medicine in a manner most extraordinary.

Whether you are a seasoned healthcare professional, a student of medicine, or simply a curious soul fascinated by the rhythms of the human body and the narratives of healing, these poems are designed to kindle your imagination and deepen your appreciation for the medical field.

Whether embarking on this journey solo or seeking a shared experience of discovery and learning with peers or loved ones, these riddles promise a fun and enriching way to enhance your understanding of medical language. From casual readers to healthcare enthusiasts, each poem offers the chance to engage your intellect and spread the joy of unlocking the secrets of medicine in a communal, interactive setting.

As you delve into each page, you will encounter terms familiar to the sphere of healthcare, transformed into poetic enigmas. From the urgency of "Cardiac Arrest" to the quiet strength in "Palliative Care," from the innovation of "Tissue Engineering" to the mystery of "Genetic Disorders," each poem is an invitation to an adventurous quest, awaiting your embarkation.

This book also acts as a bridge, linking those deeply immersed in the world of healthcare with those on the periphery. For medical professionals, it presents an opportunity to view the familiar through a fresh, more lyrical lens. For poets and dreamers, it offers a chance to uncover the poetry that resides within the precision and empathy of healthcare.

"The Healer's Verses" is more than just a book. It's a celebration of the union between the scalpel and the stanza, the diagnosis and the verse. It's an invitation to pause and reflect, to marvel at the harmony between two seemingly different realms—the world of medicine and the world of poetry.

So, embark on this unparalleled journey, where each riddle opens doors to both comprehension and amazement. Decode the intricacies of healthcare through the cadence of verse and find yourself intrigued, challenged, and inspired.

Welcome, insightful minds, to a world where science meets sonnet.

The Healer's Verses

In the realm where health and verse collide,

A curious journey, wide and wide,

"The Healer's Verses" opens the door,

To medical mysteries, lore and more.

Through the lens of rhyme, we take a peek,

At the body's wonders, unique and sleek,

Where science and art in harmony dance,

Each diagnosis given a chance.

In stanzas crafted with care and might,

Medicine's challenges brought to light,

With each riddle posed, a puzzle to solve,

In rhythmic cadence, our minds evolve.

From the heart's beat to the brain's deep thought,

Each verse a lesson, subtly taught,

Where cells and signals in verses sing,

A poetic tribute to healing's wing.

Whether you wield a stethoscope's grace,

Or simply marvel at life's steady pace,

These poems invite, with humor and flair,

To explore the depths of healthcare.

So, embark on this journey, verse by verse,

Where medicine's world, we gently traverse,

In "The Healer's Verses," find your muse,

Where code meets cadence, and insights fuse.

Riddle 1

In halls of white, I roam with care,

A healer's touch, a learned stare.

With a stethoscope, my neck adorned,

Through countless books, my mind was formed.

I diagnose, with wisdom rare,

And offer solace from despair.

In scrubs or coat, I'm often found,

Where heartbeats whisper life's profound.

A guardian of health, my creed,

To every call of need, I heed.

Not just a job, a life's pursuit,

In healing's art, I take root.

Riddle 2

With gentle hands and watchful eyes,

A caring soul in disguise.

I walk the wards from night till day,

Easing pains along the way.

A vital link in healing's chain,

In times of loss, in times of gain.

With patience vast, and heart so wide,

I stand always by your side.

Charting courses, giving meds,

Comforting hearts, fluffing beds.

A whispered prayer, a hopeful smile,

I make the journey worth the while.

Riddle 3

A fortress vast of healing's might,

Where day oft blends into the night.

Within its walls, the weary rest,

And professionals put to the test.

A beacon bright in illness' gloom,

A place where hope can find its room.

Corridors long, with stories untold,

Of battles fierce, of courage bold.

In every room, a different fight,

Against the dark, a quest for light.

Here, life begins, and sometimes ends,

A place where sorrow oft amends.

Riddle 4

A local haven, small and bright,

Where ailments meet a hopeful sight.

Not vast as some, but just as keen,

To mend the wounds that are unseen.

A doctor's care, a nurse's touch,

In this domain, they mean so much.

For ailments mild, or health's routine,

Its doors are open, its floors are clean.

A personal touch, a shorter wait,

For many, it's a gentler fate.

In every town, a beacon small,

A clinic stands, to aid all.

Riddle 5

A treasury of healing's tools,

Beyond the layman's basic schools.

Here potions, pills, and remedies,

Line shelves in vast varieties.

A guardian of compounds rare,

Dispenses care with skill to spare.

In battles against fever's might,

It offers solace through the night.

From antibiotics to creams,

It fuels the hope, the dreams, the schemes.

A crucial ally in health's quest,

Ensuring you receive the best.

Riddle 6

A chariot of urgent cries,

It speeds, it weaves, it swiftly flies.

With sirens loud and lights ablaze,

In its pursuit, time's crucial phase.

Inside, a team of ready minds,

Where skill and urgency intertwines.

A mobile haven in distress,

Aiming to save, to aid, to bless.

Through city streets or country lanes,

It carries hope, ignores the pains.

A lifeline in emergency's grasp,

A beacon hope, a safety clasp.

Riddle 7

At the crossroads of care, decisions made fast,

Where the severity's sorted, from first to last.

A pivotal point in the care that you seek,

Where the urgent are served, and the strong aid the weak.

Here, the pace is a whirl, and the stakes are high,

As professionals work, not letting time fly.

A nexus of paths, where directions are given,

To heal, to mend, and to keep the life livin'.

In this room, the journey of healing begins,

Sorting through chaos, to save those within.

A critical dance of priorities set,

Ensuring that no one's needs are left unmet.

Riddle 8

A concoction or pill, to heal or to mend,

A craft that's as old, as time's own bend.

With science and nature in tight embrace,

It battles the ills the body can face.

From herbs to compounds of complex design,

Each has a purpose, a plan, a line.

In doses measured, and effects keen,

It's the unseen warrior, oft not seen.

A silent guardian against disease's night,

Ingested in hope, in fear, in plight.

A testament to humanity's quest,

To live better lives, and put pain to rest.

Riddle 9

In the aftermath of healing's touch,

Comes a reality, that weighs much.

An enumeration of care's cost,

A tally of what's gained, what's lost.

Paper trails that follow pain,

Adding stress, to strain.

Yet within these lists, a story told,

Of services rendered, brave and bold.

A necessary evil, some would say,

For the care that came, in your dismay.

A reminder of the price of health,

And the value we place on wealth.

Riddle 10

A sweetened potion, thick and rich,

For throats that itch, a soothing switch.

In flavors varied, to ease the dose,

A liquid comfort, warmth it boasts.

Against the coughs, the colds, the flu,

It's a childhood memory, for me, for you.

A simple remedy, from the shelf,

Bringing back wellness, restoring health.

Not just a medicine, but a treat,

Making the bitter, a bit more sweet.

In every bottle, a promise kept,

To ease your ailment, with every step.

Riddle 11

A loop and pair, by ears it's worn,

To listen close to life reborn.

It hangs around the healer's neck,

To catch the sounds of heart and breath.

A tool of trade for those in white,

It whispers secrets of the fight.

Against the silence of disease,

It finds the rhythms that will please.

A bridge between the seen and heard,

Translating life without a word.

With its help, the silent speak,

Revealing truths that others seek.

Riddle 12

A brief pinch, a swift sting,

Delivering relief it will bring.

A guardian in a tiny guise,

Carrying cures of a size.

Through a needle, sharp and thin,

It battles foes that lurk within.

A liquid soldier, brave and bold,

In its journey, stories told.

Against the villains, small and vile,

It travels through the body's mile.

A moment's discomfort, for healing's gain,

A small act, to ease the pain.

Riddle 13

A silent measure of life's force,

A vital sign, a guiding course.

With cuff and gauge, it's quietly sought,

A number gained, a reading caught.

Too high or low, it whispers tales,

Of health's fine balance, when it scales.

A squeeze that hugs your arm so tight,

Revealing how you fare in fight.

This rhythm, unseen but deeply felt,

Can tell if health is sound or dealt.

A gauge of life's most vital flow,

It helps to let the healers know.

Riddle 14

Pages and files, a history told,

Of battles with heat, and wars with cold.

A chronicle kept of every ail,

Every triumph, every fail.

A treasure trove of facts so vast,

On paper, digital, meant to last.

It follows you from birth to end,

A faithful, silent, unseen friend.

In its lines, your story's kept,

Through every tear you've wept.

A guardian of your health's lore,

A key to what your future's for.

Riddle 15

A band, a tag, a simple loop,

Around your wrist, a part of the troop.

A name, a number, clearly shown,

Ensuring you're rightly known.

In a world of rush and care,

It speaks for you, when you're not there.

A silent sentinel, keeping track,

Ensuring nothing's out of whack.

In the vastness where you lay,

It's your beacon, night or day.

A small device, yet holds the key,

To your identity, so free.

Riddle 16

A chamber where the whispers tread,

On tiptoes, fighting dread.

Where monitors beep and lights blink slow,

Guarding lives in their fragile glow.

A realm where silence holds much weight,

And every moment can decide fate.

Here, the watchers keep their vigil tight,

Through the darkest hours of the night.

Each breath, each beat, under keen eyes,

Where hope and science tightly lies.

In this place, the fight's intense,

Every second holds immense sense.

Riddle 17

A portal where time races by,

Where moments breathe, live, and die.

A crossroad of fate, of pain, of fear,

Where seconds count, and help is near.

A hive of action, swift and sure,

Where skill and urgency meet the cure.

Lights flash, doors swing, the urgent call,

A haven ready for all.

Here, life's dramas unfold in haste,

No moment, no breath, goes to waste.

In this chaos, a structured dance,

Where every chance is given a chance.

Riddle 18

A box, a case, a pack so neat,

With tools to make the healing sweet.

Bandages, wipes, and antiseptic cream,

For every cut, for every scream.

A portable guardian, ready at hand,

For life's little trials that weren't planned.

In moments of need, it's there to aid,

In the battle against the pain parade.

A collection small but mighty fierce,

Bringing comfort, making tears cease.

A first response, a caring kit,

In times of trouble, a perfect fit.

Riddle 19

A promise made on paper thin,

Against the times of pain you're in.

A guardian that in silence waits,

To carry burdens, to lift the weights.

In the maze of care and cure,

It's a guide, a light, secure.

A safety net, spread wide and far,

For every wound, for every scar.

It speaks in terms of codes and claims,

A complex dance, a myriad of names.

Yet at its core, a simple aim,

To keep you safe, in health's grand game.

Riddle 20

A tiny jab, a giant leap,

Against the foes that in shadows creep.

A guardian before the battle's start,

Giving immunity, a protective art.

With science's help, a shield is made,

In hopes that sickness will fade.

A drop, a shot, so small, so slight,

Yet holds the power of healing's light.

A communal armor against the spread,

Of diseases that fill us with dread.

A proactive step, a caring act,

To keep the health of all intact.

Riddle 21

A wrap, a cover, a shield for the sore,

A hug for a wound, and so much more.

It sticks, it binds, it holds things tight,

Turning a wrong into a right.

A fabric guardian, silent and true,

Protecting the old, embracing the new.

In rolls or strips, it comes to aid,

Where cuts and scrapes are freshly made.

A simple soldier in healing's band,

Offering care with a gentle hand.

Around a finger, knee, or arm,

It works its quiet, healing charm.

Riddle 22

A sentinel of rise and fall,

In winter's chill or summer's thrall.

A mercury river, or digital read,

It tells us more than we might heed.

Beneath the tongue, or in the ear,

It measures what we often fear.

A rise too high, a drop too low,

It charts the course of health's ebb and flow.

A guardian of our inner flame,

Alerting us when illness came.

A simple tool, yet profound,

In its numbers, our wellness found.

Riddle 23

A check, a test, a thorough view,

To see if everything's working as it's due.

With taps and listens, looks and feels,

Assessing all from head to heels.

A journey through the body's land,

With a guide's knowing, gentle hand.

Eyes, ears, and mouth, all checked in turn,

For health's clear path, we all yearn.

A map is drawn of current state,

To prevent a less favorable fate.

This exploration, detailed and grand,

Ensures on solid ground, you stand.

Riddle 24

A note, a command, a healer's script,

Directions where hope and cure are crypt.

On paper penned, or digitally sent,

Its message clear, its intent meant.

A key to unlock the wellness door,

Guiding to health, and much more.

A regimen of care, laid out so plain,

In its adherence, much to gain.

Pills, liquids, to inhale or swallow,

A path to wellness, straight and narrow.

A bridge from ill to better days,

In these words, healing's ways.

Riddle 25

A chariot for those who find,

Walking straight, a task unkind.

With wheels for feet, it glides and rolls,

Aiding those with challenged strolls.

A seat of comfort, rest, and ride,

Through ups and downs, it's by your side.

In halls and paths, it makes way,

Turning obstacles into child's play.

A companion in times of need,

Supporting moves, at any speed.

Not just a tool, but freedom's wings,

In its embrace, the spirit sings.

Riddle 26

A chamber of pause, of hopes and fears,

Where minutes stretch into years.

Chairs in rows, magazines spread,

A clock ticking, time's slow tread.

Here, anticipation grows,

As the ebb of time gently flows.

Faces tell stories untold,

Waiting for news, brave and bold.

A prelude to the care within,

Where some journeys end, others begin.

A space of limbo, quiet and vast,

Holding breaths till the verdict's cast.

Riddle 27

A scheduled moment, a date with care,

Marked in calendars, prepared with flare.

A meeting set, a plan in place,

For health's concerns, a time, a space.

Not just a slot, but a promise made,

Where worries are seen, and fears fade.

A step towards wellness, a structured path,

In the diary, it marks its math.

A commitment to healing, a mutual pact,

In this time, a significant act.

A rendezvous where stories unfold,

In these moments, hope is told.

Riddle 28

A dance of skill, where blades meet flesh,

In sterile halls, life's fabric fresh.

A team in sync, with one aim in mind,

To cut away what harms, unkind.

In the theatre where silence speaks,

Each move deliberate, each outcome seeks.

Under lights bright, and drapes so clean,

A battle's fought, not always seen.

A journey through the body's maze,

Correcting errors, mending ways.

With precision, care, and art combined,

New beginnings in this space are signed.

Riddle 29

A haven post the storm's fierce rage,

A chapter next, a turning page.

Here, the weary start to mend,

On rest and care, they now depend.

Monitors beep a steady tune,

Marking progress, morning to noon.

A bridge from sleep to waking life,

A pause in the struggle, the surgical strife.

With each breath taken, strength returns,

In this room, the spirit yearns.

For health restored, for pain to cease,

In these walls, find your peace.

Riddle 30

A quest for clues, in vials so small,

Answers hidden, awaiting the call.

Blood, tissue, samples all told,

Secrets within, waiting to unfold.

Machines whir, analysts peer,

In results, the truth draws near.

A detective story of cells and genes,

Unraveling what health truly means.

Each test a step towards solving the case,

In numbers and images, a story's base.

In this pursuit, knowledge is key,

Unlocking wellness, setting it free.

Riddle 31

In shadows and light, I tell your tale,

Through bones and breaks, I never fail.

A peek inside, without a cut,

Revealing what the eyes are shut.

A silhouette of what's within,

A story of your frame, so thin.

I capture what cannot be seen,

In shades of black, white, and in between.

A guardian of secrets, deep and old,

Of tales in silence, quietly told.

With me, the hidden comes to light,

In radiant hues of night and bright.

Riddle 32

A tunnel of truth, where echoes dwell,

In magnetic tales, secrets swell.

Not just a passage, but a deep dive,

Where from your core, insights derive.

A hum, a whir, a gentle spin,

Mapping the stories kept within.

I paint with fields, not with a brush,

In silent whispers, a revealing hush.

A dance of atoms, in contrast high,

Revealing truths that do not lie.

Through me, the unseen is brought to bear,

A glimpse within, a comprehensive stare.

Riddle 33

A wave, a pulse, through liquid sent,

Reflecting back, a visual event.

Not just for those expecting joy,

But also to diagnose, not to annoy.

A screen lights up with life's first hello,

A beating heart, a gentle flow.

I speak in echoes, not in words,

In me, the song of life is heard.

A navigator through the unseen sea,

Charting courses where shadows be.

With gel and probe, I gently trace,

The outlines of a hidden face.

Riddle 34

A journey of steps, both large and small,

To regain the strength that held you tall.

With stretch and strain, and gentle motion,

I guide you back, with dedicated devotion.

A healer's hands, both firm and kind,

In every movement, hope you'll find.

Not just in muscles, but in heart,

I help piece back the broken part.

A bridge from pain to newfound strength,

With every session, we go the length.

In exercises, simple and complex,

I aim to fix what's out of specs.

Riddle 35

In a realm of white, where smiles are made,

And fears of drills somewhat fade.

A guardian of the oral gate,

Ensuring your bite is always great.

With brush and floss, I wage my fight,

Against the cavities hiding from sight.

A chair reclines, a light shines down,

In every tooth, no room for a frown.

Through checkups, cleanings, care galore,

I keep the threats of decay at bore.

In this domain, I gently tread,

Ensuring your smile's always spread.

Riddle 36

A test of sight, of light, of blur,

To find the clarity that once were.

Through lenses switched, in frames so slight,

I seek to restore your perfect sight.

A chart of letters, large to small,

I ask you to read them, one and all.

Not just a test, but a journey clear,

To bring the world to you near.

In drops and lights, I look inside,

To ensure no secrets your eyes hide.

A guardian of vision, so keen,

Ensuring all beauty is seen.

Riddle 37

A visit planned, with health in mind,

To leave no hidden ailment behind.

A thorough look, from head to toe,

Ensuring wellness continues to flow.

With stethoscope, and gentle prod,

I seek to find what odds are odd.

A conversation, a test or two,

To ensure you're fit, through and through.

In this routine, a peace of mind,

In preventive care, relief we find.

A yearly ritual, so it seems,

To chase away the ill-health dreams.

Riddle 38

A comprehensive review, a detailed scan,

To catch the issues before they span.

Blood and pressure, weight and height,

Evaluated to ensure you're right.

A holistic view, of body and mind,

Seeking to leave no stone unturned, no bind.

A preventative measure, so wise,

Spotting troubles before they rise.

In labs and chats, insights we gain,

To keep you on the healthiest plane.

A pledge to wellbeing, broad and deep,

A commitment to your wellness we keep.

Riddle 39

A prick, a jab, a tiny bite,

In your arm, to make things right.

A shield against the viral spread,

Keeping you out of the sickbed.

Each year anew, a formula made,

In hopes your immunity won't fade.

A little discomfort, for a lot of gain,

In this battle against the flu strain.

A seasonal ally, in a syringe small,

Offering protection for one and all.

In this act, so quick and sharp,

We aim to play a preventive harp.

Riddle 40

A guide in the maze of food and diet,

Offering wisdom, you should try it.

Not just what, but how and when,

Teaching you the nutritional zen.

With plans and charts, a path we weave,

Towards the health goals you conceive.

In the jungle of carbs, fats, and protein,

I light the way, keeping it lean.

A counselor, a coach, in eating right,

Helping your wellness reach new height.

In every meal, a choice to make,

I'm here to help, for your health's sake.

Riddle 41

A healer for the young, the small,

Who treats the tiny tots who crawl.

With gentle hands and soothing voice,

Makes little hearts and souls rejoice.

From bumps to fevers, coughs to cries,

Under their watchful care, health lies.

They chart the growth, the leaps, the bounds,

Ensuring wellness all around.

With stickers, smiles, a playful chat,

They make no child afraid of that.

A guardian of childhood's bloom,

Ensuring life can safely zoom.

Riddle 42

A specialist in women's care,

With knowledge deep, and manner fair.

Through every phase of life's grand tour,

They guide, they help, and much ensure.

From youth to age, in times of change,

They navigate the wide and strange.

In their hands, life's mysteries unfold,

With compassion and courage bold.

A partner in health, a confidant true,

For the many, not just the few.

Ensuring wellness, comfort, trust,

In their care, you're more than just.

Riddle 43

A master of the bone and joint,

With skills that never disappoint.

From fractures, sprains, to chronic pain,

They strive to make you whole again.

With casts and braces, therapy's guide,

They're by your side, stride for stride.

A sculptor of the human frame,

Restoring movement, quelling flame.

In their realm, mobility's king,

To every patient hope they bring.

Through surgery or rehab's path,

They lead the way, they clear the wrath.

Riddle 44

A navigator of the mind,

In their care, peace you'll find.

With words, with meds, a balanced hand,

They help the lost to understand.

The inner workings, deep and vast,

They untangle webs that are cast.

In the realm of thought and dream,

They light the way, a guiding beam.

A healer of the mental strife,

They work to bring back quality of life.

In sessions long or short, they seek,

To strengthen minds, make strong the weak.

Riddle 45

Within your walls, the care comes to you,

A helping hand in what you go through.

For recovery, age, or special need,

They're there to help, to guide, to lead.

A presence kind, a touch so light,

Making burdens seem less tight.

From dawn till dusk, or through the night,

They ensure everything's alright.

Not just a service, but a friend,

On whom you can depend.

In comfort of your own abode,

They lighten your every load.

Riddle 46

A community where care is key,

For those in life's late symphony.

With staff to aid, both night and day,

They ensure well-being in every way.

A place of rest, of care, of peace,

Where worries and pains can cease.

Activities, meals, and friendships bloom,

Dispelling loneliness and gloom.

Here, the golden years shine bright,

With every need brought into light.

A harbor safe, a caring space,

Where every soul finds its grace.

Riddle 47

Tiny guardians in a jar,

Boosting health, both near and far.

A, B, C, and D,

In their presence, wellness be.

From sun, from soil, from food, from sea,

They come to help you be the best you can be.

Essential for growth, for life, for glow,

They're more important than you might know.

Daily doses, colors bright,

Filling gaps, making right.

In chew, in pill, in liquid's pour,

They're part of health's core lore.

Riddle 48

A warrior against unseen foes,

Where it flows, safety grows.

On surfaces, skin, in every nook,

It cleanses with just a single look.

Bacteria, viruses, meet their doom,

In its presence, they can't bloom.

A scent of clean, a touch of care,

Leaving behind fresh, pure air.

In bottle, wipe, or aerosol form,

Against the swarm, it's far from norm.

A protector in every space,

Ensuring germs leave no trace.

Riddle 49

In the palm of your hand, a tool so bright,

Tracking wellness, day and night.

Steps and sleep, heart rate, too,

It keeps an eye on all you do.

Reminders for meds, hydration's nudge,

On your health, it won't budge.

A personal coach, a guide, a friend,

Supporting your health journey to the end.

Data collected, insights gained,

Towards a healthier life, aimed.

In tech we trust, in apps we see,

A future of wellness, handy and free.

Riddle 50

A chill embrace for bumps and aches,

A soothing touch that never fakes.

In freezer it waits, for its time to shine,

Bringing relief, by design.

Swelling and pain, it gently fights,

Turning discomfort into delights.

Flexible, ready, cold and nice,

It's a simple, effective, icy device.

Wrap it up, and lay it down,

On your face, remove that frown.

A frosty friend in times of need,

Offering comfort, at lightning speed.

Riddle 51

A quest to find what lurks within,

That makes your eyes water, your head spin.

A prick, a scratch, a tiny spot,

Reveals the foes that you've got.

In rows they sit upon your skin,

Waiting for reactions to begin.

A map to navigate your sneeze,

To give you comfort and ease.

Not a treasure hunt for gold,

But for answers clear and bold.

This test, a guide through sneezy mists,

Helps you find what your body resists.

Riddle 52

A gift of life, from vein to vein,

A simple act, a gainful gain.

In chairs reclined, arms outstretched wide,

You give so others may abide.

A pint, a bag, a liquid red,

Carries hope for those who dread.

A chain of life, link by link,

More vital than you might think.

Not just a deed of noble heart,

But a science, an art.

For every drop that you afford,

Brings strength restored, life accorded.

Riddle 53

A whisperer of sounds so slight,

Transforming silence into light.

A tiny device, discreetly worn,

Bringing melodies that were torn.

It captures, amplifies the breeze,

The chatter of leaves, the hum of bees.

Not just a tool, but a key,

To unlock the world's symphony.

In its circuitry, sounds are found,

And life's volume turns around.

A companion in your auditory quest,

Ensuring you hear life's best.

Riddle 54

A guardian against the day's bright glare,

A lotion, a cream, with care to spare.

It shields your skin from fiery foe,

Ensuring you're not the sun's aglow.

With SPF as its sword,

It battles rays, largely ignored.

Applied in layers, light or thick,

It keeps the skin from getting sick.

Not just a summer's passing friend,

But a year-round guard to defend.

In its protection, safely bask,

For it performs a crucial task.

Riddle 55

A warrior in a bottle, clear,

Fighting germs far and near.

On cuts, on scrapes, it's bravely spread,

Killing bacteria, ensuring they're dead.

A sting, perhaps, a sign it's there,

Cleaning wounds with utmost care.

Not just a cleaner, but a guard,

In healing's journey, a vital card.

It fights in silence, battles unseen,

Ensuring that your wounds are clean.

A first aid hero, without a cape,

Securing health in its liquid shape.

Riddle 56

A lozenge of relief, a soothing balm,

For throats that ache, a peaceful calm.

Wrapped in wrappers, small and neat,

Each one a treat to meet defeat.

With menthol's chill, or honey's hug,

They quell the cough, a stubborn bug.

Not just a candy, but a cure,

For symptoms that you might endure.

In pockets, purses, they're carried around,

Ready to soothe without a sound.

A simple remedy, tried and true,

They offer comfort, through and through.

Riddle 57

A gathering of wellness, under tents so wide,

Where advice and screenings calmly abide.

From booth to booth, you wander and learn,

About health's treasures at every turn.

A festival of care, free and fair,

Offering insights on how to repair.

With tests, with talks, with tools to try,

They aim to keep your spirits high.

Not just an event, but a communal dare,

To take charge of your health, to be aware.

A carnival of sorts, without the rides,

Promoting wellness, where guidance resides.

Riddle 58

A lifeline in straps, clear and snug,

Breathing life with each tug.

Above the clouds or in care's embrace,

It delivers breath at a steady pace.

A cascade of air, pure and sweet,

Making every inhalation a treat.

Not just a mask, but a vital friend,

In moments when you need to mend.

In emergencies, it's first to descend,

Offering oxygen, a helping hand to lend.

A bearer of life's essential flow,

Ensuring vitality continues to grow.

Riddle 59

A band of insight, worn on the wrist,

Counting steps, sleep, and when you twist.

It watches, records, day and night,

Guiding you towards a healthier plight.

With every beat of your heart, it's aware,

Tracking progress, how much you dare.

Not just a watch, but a coach so tight,

Encouraging moves, out of sight.

It vibrates for attention, nudges to move,

In the dance of wellness, it helps you groove.

A digital companion in fitness quests,

Ensuring you're meeting all your bests.

Riddle 60

A whisper of caution, worn on the arm,

A sentinel of safety, to protect from harm.

In silver or gold, or hues discreet,

It speaks when you might not, so sweet.

Engraved with wisdom, for eyes to see,

Informing helpers of the key.

Allergies, conditions, in short, it tells,

A story of caution, where significance dwells.

Not just jewelry, but a lifeline's part,

In moments critical, it plays its part.

A bearer of tales, in silence it waits,

Guarding the wearer from unforeseen fates.

Riddle 61

A map of life, beneath the skin,

Where tales of us all begin.

Bones and muscles, veins in thrall,

A blueprint detailed, encompassing all.

With every layer, deeper we dive,

Exploring where our mysteries thrive.

From head to toe, each part we name,

In this complex, bodily game.

A study of structure, so vast, so grand,

On this foundation, we understand.

Not just a subject, but a guide,

To the wonders that inside us hide.

Riddle 62

The study of life, in action seen,

How we breathe, grow, and glean.

A tale of cells, of heart, of lung,

Of every process, unsung.

How blood flows, how we feel the heat,

The rhythm of life, in every beat.

A science of functions, systems, might,

Revealing how we fight our fight.

In this field, we come to know,

How life's currents ebb and flow.

Not just mechanics, but the art,

Of body's symphony, part by part.

Riddle 63

A tale of when things go awry,

Under the microscope, truths lie.

Disease and disorder, cells at war,

Revealing what's hidden, in the core.

A detective story, of sorts, you see,

Deciphering illness's mystery.

In tissues and samples, answers found,

To why health's balance is not sound.

The study of sickness, in depth, in detail,

On this quest, we sail, we trail.

Not just a science, but a key,

Unlocking cures, setting us free.

Riddle 64

A realm of potions, of pills, of cure,

Where remedies and treatments endure.

The study of drugs, in body's maze,

How they heal, or sedate, or amaze.

From herb to synthetic, in trials, in tests,

Seeking to offer their very best.

How compounds interact, side by side,

In this knowledge, we confide.

A bridge between science and healing's touch,

In this field, we owe so much.

Not merely drugs, but hope in a dose,

In pharmacology, relief we diagnose.

Riddle 65

A sample taken, a piece so small,

Under the lens, it tells us all.

A quest for truth, in tissue's tale,

Seeking answers, without fail.

Is it benign, or something feared?

In these cells, the future's peered.

A bridge between doubt and knowing's light,

Guiding us through health's night.

Not just a procedure, but a quest,

In its results, our fears laid to rest.

A small piece, a vast insight,

In biopsy, we find our fight.

Riddle 66

The realm of the heart, its beat, its sound,

In its rhythm, life is found.

A study of vessels, of blood, of flow,

Of how love's metaphor can literally show.

From thump to murmur, in echo's tale,

Cardiology seeks to unveil.

A pulse of life, in every beat,

Ensuring our ticker's defeat.

Not just a specialty, but a core,

In this science, life's secrets pour.

A guardian of beats, of life, of song,

In cardiology, hearts stay strong.

Riddle 67

The network vast, of nerve and cell,

Where thoughts and dreams and feelings dwell.

A study of brain, of spine, of cord,

In its complexities, wonders stored.

From twitch to thought, from pain to play,

In neurology's realm, we find our way.

A puzzle of neurons, in connection's dance,

Unlocking the mysteries of mind's expanse.

Not just a field, but a frontier,

Where the essence of being comes near.

In the study of nerves, a discovery vast,

In neurology, the die is cast.

Riddle 68

A battle waged, in cells gone wild,

Seeking to tame what's been reviled.

A study of cancer, its forms, its might,

In oncology, we find our fight.

With treatments, research, a hope to cure,

For patients, a future to ensure.

In tumors' shadow, a light is sought,

With every lesson, hard fought.

Not just a specialty, but a quest,

To offer those afflicted, the very best.

A field of care, of hope, of life,

In oncology, we cut through strife.

Riddle 69

A realm where young ones find their voice,

In health and sickness, a specialty's choice.

From newborn cries to adolescent woes,

Pediatrics watches as each child grows.

With gentle hands and hearts so big,

They dance a care-filled, life-giving jig.

Vaccines, check-ups, growth and more,

In their care, children's health they restore.

Not just a field, but a joyful task,

In their dedication, we bask.

A protector of youth, of laugh, of tear,

In pediatrics, young lives we revere.

Riddle 70

The landscape of mind, complex and deep,

Where shadows linger, and sorrows weep.

A study of psyche, of emotion, of care,

In psychiatry, healing's share.

From stress to sorrow, from anxiety to fear,

It offers a space for healing to steer.

With words, with therapy, with a listening ear,

It seeks to make mental troubles clear.

Not just a practice, but a profound art,

Where understanding is only the start.

In the care of the soul, a delicate might,

In psychiatry, we find the light.

Riddle 71

Through beams and waves, I see within,

A world of shadow, bone, and skin.

Not with eyes, but with machines,

I reveal what unseen means.

From chest to limb, in detail fine,

I make the invisible, brilliantly shine.

In my realm, no secret hides,

Every shadow, truth abides.

A picture worth more than words can say,

In shades of gray, life's display.

Not just an image, but a key,

To unlock health's mystery.

Riddle 72

A study of shields, of body's fight,

Against invaders, day and night.

Tiny warriors, vast and keen,

Guarding scenes unseen.

In blood and tissue, they stand guard,

Their vigilance, our reward.

Vaccines, allergies, in their domain,

In their balance, health we gain.

A complex dance of cell and gene,

Where harmony is the unseen scene.

Not just science, but life's own lore,

Guarding well-being, forevermore.

Riddle 73

A canvas vast, of hue and texture,

Your skin's the subject of my lecture.

From rash to wrinkle, mole to scar,

I study blemishes, near and far.

The largest organ, openly seen,

Its health and woes, what they mean.

In lotions, lasers, knowledge deep,

Your skin's well-being, I seek to keep.

Not just the surface, but below,

Where cells and stories grow.

A field of care, both art and science,

In skin's health, we place reliance.

Riddle 74

A whisper network, silent, vast,

Hormones, the cast, from first to last.

They signal, regulate, and guide,

In their balance, well-being resides.

From thyroid's hum to insulin's dance,

They shape our growth, sleep, and trance.

A detective's work, in essence, mine,

Seeking clues in every sign.

Not just glands, but life's own rhythm,

In their flow, health's prism.

A specialty, both broad and deep,

In hormone's song, wellness we reap.

Riddle 75

A journey through the inner tube,

Digestion's maze, and nutrient's cube.

From mouth to gut, in peristalsis' wave,

I study how food behaves.

Ulcers, reflux, and diseases crohn,

In my field, they're well known.

With scope and screen, I explore deep,

Ensuring your digestive keep.

Not just a tract, but a complex lane,

Where health's balance, we ascertain.

A field of care, with insights vast,

In your gut's health, a lasting cast.

Riddle 76

The study of blood, in cells and flow,

In its stream, life's glow.

Red and white, platelets too,

Each has its job, its cue.

Anemia, clotting, and cancers rare,

Under my gaze, I lay them bare.

In veins and marrow, secrets kept,

Through my knowledge, insights lept.

Not just fluid, but a vital stream,

Carrying oxygen, nutrients, a dream.

A specialty deep, with care so bold,

In blood's tale, life's told.

Riddle 77

The keepers of fluid, filters fine,

Kidneys' work, in their design.

From toxin removal to balance of salt,

In their health, life's vault.

Dialysis, stones, and hypertension's call,

In my care, I address them all.

A study of function, of renal flair,

Ensuring your filters are in repair.

Not just organs, but life's purifiers,

In their health, the body's desires.

A field of deep care and insight,

In kidney's health, we fight the fight.

Riddle 78

A guardian of birth, of life's first cry,

In my hands, new beginnings lie.

From conception's dawn to labor's end,

On my care, lives depend.

Monitoring growth, ensuring health,

In this journey, life's greatest wealth.

A specialty of joy, of hope's embrace,

Welcoming new life, into our space.

Not just a practice, but a sacred art,

In life's start, I play my part.

A field of miracles, day by day,

In obstetrics, life finds its way.

Riddle 79

A caretaker of women, through every stage,

From youth, to maturity, to age.

In wellness and woe, in health's ebb and flow,

I guide, advise, and knowledge bestow.

A specialty deep, with a focus so true,

On women's health, in all its hue.

From preventive care to problems deep,

In my care, their well-being I keep.

Not just a doctor, but a trusted guide,

In women's health, I take pride.

A field of care, vast and profound,

In gynecology, solutions are found.

Riddle 80

A seer of sights, of light, of blink,

In eye's health, deeper I think.

From vision sharp to blindness' brink,

I study all, in eye's link.

Glasses, surgery, diseases rare,

In my gaze, I lay them bare.

A guardian of the visual soul,

Ensuring sight's a goal.

Not just a practice, but a craft,

In vision's care, we're never daft.

A field of focus, precision, care,

In ophthalmology, vision we repair.

Riddle 81

In the realm where bones and joints unite,

A craft that sets the crooked right.

When limbs are fractured, tendons torn,

In my care, they're reborn.

From spine to ankle, hip to wrist,

I mend the framework that you've missed.

A cast, a brace, a surgery fine,

Restoring movement, line by line.

Not just bones, but lives I fix,

With tools and skills in my mix.

A healer of the framework's woes,

Ensuring on your feet, you rose.

Riddle 82

A keeper of the gates of speech,

Where air and sound together reach.

Ears, nose, throat, my domain vast,

Ensuring your senses last.

Sinus whispers, hearing's loss,

Tonsils' troubles, I come across.

With scope and light, I peer inside,

To find what ailments may reside.

Not just a doctor, but a guide,

In health's journey, by your side.

A specialist of head and neck,

Ensuring you're in check.

Riddle 83

In the breath of life, my focus lies,

Where air flows in, and spirit flies.

The whisper of lungs, both large and small,

I listen to their every call.

Asthma's wheeze, pneumonia's cough,

In their cure, I'm not soft.

With tests and scans, I seek to find,

The secrets that in breath are twined.

Not just organs, but life's essence,

In their health, my presence.

A guardian of the air you breathe,

Ensuring from no ailment you seethe.

Riddle 84

A detective in the realm of ache,

Where joints and muscles protests make.

Arthritis' grip, lupus' stealth,

In their mysteries, I find wealth.

With needle and lab, I search for clues,

To offer patients relief, not blues.

Inflammation's trail, I keenly follow,

To bring back days bright, not hollow.

Not just a practitioner, but a sleuth,

Seeking the pathways to health, to truth.

A healer of the body's silent cries,

Ensuring your spirit again, it flies.

Riddle 85

A guardian of the liquid flow,

Where waters of life ceaselessly go.

Kidneys, bladder, in their charge,

Ensuring their pathways, large.

Stones and streams, infections' fight,

In my care, they're brought to light.

With skill and science, I navigate,

To keep the flow unobstructate.

Not just a doctor, but a guide,

Ensuring healthily you'll bide.

A specialist of the water's course,

Ensuring it runs without force.

Riddle 86

In the realm of sleep, induced and deep,

Where pain is silenced, in a leap.

With gases and drugs, I tenderly weave,

A slumber for those about to receive.

A guardian at the edge of dreams,

Ensuring peace, no matter what seams.

In operations' silent creed,

I stand by, in your need.

Not just a bringer of night's embrace,

But a watcher, ensuring a safe space.

In my hands, your trust is kept,

Ensuring by pain, you're not swept.

Riddle 87

In the whirlwind of the unforeseen,

Where moments are critical, and margins lean.

I stand ready, day and night,

To turn health's battles, into light.

With swift action and decisive care,

I navigate the medical scare.

Not just a doctor, but a rapid force,

Ensuring health's on its course.

A master of the urgent and the acute,

Ensuring dangers, we refute.

In life's most sudden, stark alarms,

I welcome you with open arms.

Riddle 88

A guardian of health, for young and old,

In my care, your life's story's told.

From first breaths to the golden years,

I'm with you through joys and tears.

Vaccines, check-ups, counsel wise,

In your family's health, my heart lies.

Not just a physician, but a friend,

On whom for lifelong care, you depend.

A tapestry of health, I weave,

Ensuring wellness, you achieve.

In the fabric of community and home,

I ensure you're never alone.

Riddle 89

In the autumn of life, my care's bestowed,

Ensuring golden years in health are owed.

With patience and wisdom, I tenderly guide,

Ensuring age's ailments don't abide.

Memory's fog, bones that creak,

For their relief, it's me they seek.

Not just a doctor, but a gentle hand,

Helping you withstand time's sand.

A specialist in the art of aging,

Ensuring life's book, you're still paging.

In the care of those with stories told,

I ensure they're bold, not cold.

Riddle 90

A sleuth in the realm of microscopic foes,

Where bacteria and viruses propose.

With vaccines, antibiotics, my toolkit's prepared,

To confront the outbreaks, as I've dared.

Ebola, flu, or COVID's strain,

In my battle, I sustain.

Not just a doctor, but a global guard,

Ensuring pandemics, we retard.

A healer in the fight against the spread,

Ensuring health's tapestry is widely spread.

In the war against invisible threats,

I stand vigilant, with no regrets.

Riddle 91

In a realm where whispers tread lightly on air,

And monitors sing in a rhythm of care.

Here, vigilance reigns, both day and night,

Guarding lives with all our might.

A haven for those at edge, so dire,

Where hope and skill conspire.

Each breath, each beat, under watchful eyes,

Where expertise and compassion rise.

Not just a place, but a critical dance,

Giving every soul a fighting chance.

In this space, the critical speak,

In the language of the strong, not weak.

Riddle 92

A code of life, in twists and folds,

Secrets within, each strand holds.

From parent to child, the tales are passed,

In the dance of genes, vast.

A story of you, written so deep,

In DNA's keep.

Diseases, traits, in patterns told,

A future's outline, bold.

Not just a science, but a map to guide,

In genetic streams, we confide.

Unlocking mysteries of the familial tie,

In our code, answers lie.

Riddle 93

After the storm, when damage is done,

A journey of healing, has just begun.

With patience and strength, we find our way,

Restoring what was lost, in day by day.

A practice in hope, in recovery's art,

Teaching bodies to again, start.

Not just the physical, but mind and soul,

In holistic care, we find our goal.

A bridge from injury back to life,

Reducing pain, easing strife.

In every step, a victory small,

In rehabilitation, we reclaim it all.

Riddle 94

In the arena where athletes strive,

Keeping dreams and bodies alive.

A study in motion, in stress and strain,

In pursuit of victory, in joy and pain.

From tendon to muscle, to joint and bone,

Ensuring strength, not alone.

A guardian against the wear and tear,

Offering care, beyond compare.

Not just for the elite, but for all in motion,

In sports medicine, we pour our devotion.

Keeping you running, jumping, in play,

In healthful spirit, every day.

Riddle 95

A tale of two, hidden within,

One brings joy, the other sin.

A waxy substance, friend and foe,

Through your blood, it may freely flow.

In balance, a vital part of life,

In excess, it brings strife.

A marker of health, unseen, untold,

In its levels, stories unfold.

Not just a number to be feared or fought,

But a balance, wisely sought.

In diet, in exercise, it finds its place,

In the dance of health, it has its space.

Riddle 96

A silent tale of sugar and blood,

Where balance lost, becomes a flood.

In cells hungry, in energy spent,

A body's harmony, bent.

A vigilant watch, day and night,

To keep the levels just right.

Not just a word, but a life's rewrite,

In this challenge, a constant fight.

With care, with knowledge, the tide we turn,

In lessons of health, we learn.

A story of many, young and old,

In whispers of warning, bold.

Riddle 97

A line, a spike, a valley, a loop,

Tales of the heart, in a group.

A rhythm captured on paper, so stark,

Each beat, a life's mark.

Not just squiggles, but a heart's song,

In its rhythm, right or wrong.

A diagnostic dance, precise and keen,

In its traces, life's seen.

A graph of life, in beats and pauses,

In its lines, a story causes.

A silent language, speaking loud,

In ECG, heart's story, proud.

Riddle 98

In a tunnel of sound, a magnetic hum,

Revealing secrets, otherwise mum.

Not with light, but fields so strong,

Creating pictures, detailed and long.

A journey inside, without a cut,

Each layer, each structure, but.

Not just an image, but a deep insight,

In shades of grey, black, and white.

A window to the inner self,

In health's quest, a valuable wealth.

A marvel of science, in detail, it sings,

In MRI, the body's inner rings.

Riddle 99

A warrior small, against the swarm,

In battles unseen, they perform.

Against the invaders, they stand tall,

Saving lives, big and small.

Not just a pill, but a shield in fight,

In darkness, they bring light.

A legacy of wonder, from mold and earth,

In their power, rebirth.

A careful use, a guarded might,

Ensuring health's right.

In this arsenal against disease's night,

Antibiotics, our knight.

Riddle 100

A wave that spreads, far and wide,

Where caution and fear coincide.

Not just a sickness, but a spread,

In numbers and shadows, dread.

A challenge to health, to society's weave,

In our response, what we achieve.

A test of systems, of humanity's care,

In the face of crisis, what we dare.

Not just a moment, but a history's mark,

In its wake, a change, stark.

A call to arms, in science and heart,

In overcoming, we all have a part.

Riddle 101

A shadow that crosses borders unseen,

Touching lives, where it's been.

A whisper that grows into a roar,

Changing what we knew before.

It travels without passport or visa,

From bustling cities to the calm of Pisa.

A test of our will, our care, our might,

In darkness, seeking out the light.

Not just a sickness, but a global call,

To stand together, one and all.

A lesson in unity, in health's precious worth,

Reminding us of what we cherish on Earth.

Riddle 102

In the lab where art and science blend,

Creating solutions, mend by mend.

From devices that listen to hearts that beat,

To bionic limbs that move so neat.

A bridge between the possible and dreams,

Turning silent screams into beams.

A craft where life's puzzles are pieced together,

With innovation that's light as a feather.

Not just invention, but hope's design,

In every creation, a lifeline.

A meld of minds, in quest to heal,

Where science meets compassion, real.

Riddle 103

In the realm where data dances with care,

Turning numbers into a healthful affair.

A digital symphony of records and stats,

Helping doctors combat health combats.

From bytes and bits, insights are born,

Making sure no warning is torn.

A nexus of technology and healing's art,

Ensuring medicine plays its part.

Not just information, but a guiding light,

In the quest for wellness, day and night.

A field where knowledge is power, truly said,

In its flow, health's future is read.

Riddle 104

Across the wires, a doctor's face,

Bringing care to the most remote place.

A consultation without a room,

From comfort of home, dispelling gloom.

A click, a call, a screen away,

Health advice, any time of day.

Breaking barriers, distances no more,

Opening up a virtual door.

Not just a visit, but a connection made,

Where healing's offered, fears allayed.

A modern twist to ancient creed,

In technology, a new way to heed.

Riddle 105

A journey of discovery, step by step,

Where hypotheses are keenly kept.

From theory to therapy, the path is long,

Testing what's right, avoiding what's wrong.

Participants and researchers, hand in hand,

Seeking to understand, to expand.

A crucible of innovation, under watchful eyes,

Where safety and efficacy are the prize.

Not just experiments, but hope in trial,

In each phase, a mile.

A bridge from bench to bedside, where,

New treatments emerge, fair and square.

Riddle 106

The building blocks of life, so potent, so small,

Holding the power to change, to enthrall.

From these cells, new tissues can grow,

Healing wounds, making life's flow.

A promise of regeneration, so vast,

In their potential, a future cast.

Not just cells, but a fountain of youth,

In their division, lies a profound truth.

A frontier in medicine, so bold,

Where the mysteries of life unfold.

In their essence, a new way to heal,

A canvas blank, for science to reveal.

Riddle 107

In the code of life, a letter's change,

Can make the ordinary, strange.

But with precision, we enter the fray,

Correcting genes, in a new way.

A vector, a carrier, a change so small,

With the power to rewrite, to enthrall.

Not just treatment, but transformation,

Offering hope, a new foundation.

A leap into genetics' deepest sea,

Where we edit life's recipe.

A bold approach to maladies old,

In gene therapy, the future's told.

Riddle 108

A peek inside, with minimal mark,

Illuminating the inner dark.

With lens and light, through portals small,

Exploring mysteries, one and all.

A lessened pain, a quicker mend,

On this technique, patients depend.

Not just a procedure, but a vision clear,

Reducing the recovery, and the fear.

A minimal invasion, a maximal gain,

In this approach, less is the pain.

A revolution in surgery's art,

Where healing's quicker to start.

Riddle 109

A craft where science and hope intertwine,

Offering movement, design so fine.

From limbs that were lost, to hands that grasp,

Innovation's embrace, a future to clasp.

Not just replacements, but freedom regained,

In every creation, life's sustained.

A blend of engineering, compassion, and skill,

Making sure life's hurdles, we still fulfill.

Not just devices, but extensions of will,

In prosthetics, dreams we instill.

A testament to human spirit's quest,

In overcoming, we find our best.

Riddle 110

A guardian so small, against foes unseen,

Teaching our bodies, keeping them keen.

A pinch, a jab, a moment's discomfort,

For a shield that's life's consort.

Not just prevention, but a promise kept,

Through years and tears, adept.

A fight against the viral tide,

In this science, we confide.

A triumph of research, care, and hope,

Giving us with threats, a way to cope.

Not just an injection, but life's defense,

In vaccines, we find resilience intense.

Riddle 111

A thief in the night, taking what's red,

Leaving you tired, weak, in bed.

Not enough soldiers to carry the fight,

Your energy stolen, with all its might.

A craving for ice, a breathless sigh,

Underneath a pale sky.

Iron, B12, might be the key,

To bring back strength to thee.

Not just a condition of the blood,

But a battle, a nutritional flood.

A quest for more, inside your vein,

To feel yourself, whole again.

Riddle 112

A wheeze, a cough, a struggle for air,

An invisible squeeze, hardly fair.

Triggers abound, in fur, in pollen,

Your chest feels tight, all swollen.

A rescue inhaler, your faithful friend,

On which, for breath, you depend.

Not just an ailment of the lung,

But a melody, unsung.

A battle for breath, day and night,

Seeking air, with all your might.

A condition, not just a wheeze or gasp,

In its grasp, for freedom, you clasp.

Riddle 113

A spectrum wide, where minds dance free,

Seeing the world differently, with glee.

Words and social cues, a different song,

Where unique perspectives belong.

A puzzle piece, not quite the same,

In a picture broader, than its frame.

Not less, not more, but varied in tune,

Under the same sun and moon.

A challenge in connecting, side by side,

In their own time, they confide.

A condition, not a disease to cure,

In their world, pure and sure.

Riddle 114

A rollercoaster of emotion, high and low,

In rapid succession, they come and go.

Euphoria's peak, despair's deep dive,

Struggling within, to stay alive.

Not just mood swings, but more profound,

In their extremes, they're bound.

A quest for balance, in the mind's sea,

Seeking stability, a plea.

A condition, a challenge, day by day,

In their world, shades of gray.

Not just a label, but a life's story,

In their journey, moments of glory.

Riddle 115

A challenge in movement, coordination, and grace,

In muscles and nerves, an ongoing race.

Not a disease, but a condition at birth,

Affecting actions, for all they're worth.

A spectrum wide, with varying degree,

In each, a strength, a plea.

A quest for independence, in each task,

In support and understanding, they bask.

Not just a limitation, but a different way,

To explore the world, every day.

A condition, not defining, but part,

Of their journey, from the start.

Riddle 116

A thief of memories, subtle and sly,

Stealing the past, as days go by.

A fog that thickens, obscuring the mind,

Leaving fragments of life behind.

Not just forgetfulness, but deeper still,

A challenge of will.

A journey backward, in time's own flow,

Struggling to remember, to know.

A condition, a trial, not just of age,

But a battle, on a different stage.

Not just a loss, but a change in being,

In their eyes, a different seeing.

Riddle 117

A shadow that dims, the brightest day,

A weight that pulls, come what may.

Not just sadness, but a deeper trench,

In its grip, the soul clenches.

A silent scream, a hidden tear,

A battle with an unseen fear.

A quest for light, in the dark,

A spark of hope, to embark.

A condition, not just of mind, but soul,

In its journey, to become whole.

Not just a phase, but a fight,

In the darkness, seeking light.

Riddle 118

A storm within, unexpected, fierce,

Where consciousness seems to pierce.

A seizure's grip, sudden and swift,

In the brain's tide, adrift.

Not just a moment, but a lifelong quest,

In understanding, rest.

A condition of the brain, complex and vast,

In its mystery, cast.

Not just an ailment, but a part of life,

In its unpredictability, strife.

A journey of care, of knowledge, of hope,

In its challenges, we cope.

Riddle 119

A silent alarm, in the night, it may call,

A chest's heavy weight, a fall.

Not just a pain, but a warning sign,

Of a heart struggling, in line.

A blockage, a clot, a narrowed path,

Leading to aftermath.

A wake-up call, to heed, to act,

In lifestyle, a pact.

Not just an event, but a life changed,

Priorities rearranged.

A reminder of mortality, so stark,

In health's journey, a mark.

Riddle 120

A silent pressure, rising unseen,

In vessels deep, not keen.

A force against the walls, so strong,

Where blood's flow doesn't belong.

Not just numbers, but a risk, untold,

In its grip, bold.

A condition of stealth, without a sign,

In its presence, align.

A call to care, to monitor, to change,

In lifestyle, rearrange.

Not just a diagnosis, but a life's quest,

In its challenge, do your best.

Riddle 121

A silent challenge, a couple's test,

Where hopes and dreams refuse to rest.

A journey long, with ups and downs,

Faced with smiles, met with frowns.

Not just a path of physical toll,

But a deep quest of the soul.

In labs and clinics, answers sought,

With love and science, battles fought.

A struggle hidden, often unseen,

In pursuit of a family dream.

Not merely absence, but a quest for life,

Together, through the strife.

Riddle 122

A silent war within the blood,

Where cells rebel, a flood.

Not just a battle, but a siege inside,

Seeking health, far and wide.

A challenge of the marrow's might,

In shadows, seeking light.

With strength and courage, the fight is met,

In hope and care, the path is set.

A journey through uncertainty's door,

With resilience, hearts soar.

Not just a disease, but a life's test,

In bravery, stories are expressed.

Riddle 123

A shadow lurking, skin's betray,

Under the sun's deceptive ray.

A mark that changes, grows, and spreads,

In silent whispers, fear treads.

Not just a spot, but a warning clear,

Prompting action, overcoming fear.

A battle on the surface fought,

In early detection, safety sought.

A challenge met, with vigilance and care,

In awareness, lives we spare.

Not merely a condition of the skin,

But a reminder of the fight within.

Riddle 124

A storm within, a rapid onset,

Where fever, headache, and fear beset.

A cloak of pain around the brain,

Seeking solace, relief in vain.

Not just an illness, but a race against time,

In every symptom, a mountain to climb.

A test of will, of medicine's might,

In darkness, searching for light.

A battle fierce, with outcomes unknown,

In unity, strength is shown.

Not merely an infection's claim,

But a reminder of life's fragile flame.

Riddle 125

A thief in the night, stealing strength unseen,

Leaving behind what once had been.

Bones whispering, brittle and frail,

A tale of loss, a silent wail.

Not just a weakening, but a silent call,

Prompting action, before a fall.

A challenge of diet, exercise, and care,

In prevention, hope we share.

A test of time, of body's reserve,

In its message, a purpose to serve.

Not merely an age's sign,

But a quest for health, to redefine.

Riddle 126

A tremor, a shake, a slow steal of grace,

A battle within, a determined pace.

Not just a movement, but a life rearranged,

Within limitations, worlds exchanged.

A challenge in every step, every task,

In support and love, we bask.

A journey through trembles and time,

With courage, a mountain to climb.

Not just a disease, but a story told,

In every heart, bravery bold.

Not merely a condition's name,

But a testament to the human flame.

Riddle 127

A sudden storm, a brain under siege,

Where time and response, must converge.

Not just a moment, but a life changed,

In an instant, worlds rearranged.

A test of strength, of will, of heart,

In recovery, a new start.

A journey through rehab, through care,

In every effort, hope we share.

Not just an event, but a path anew,

With resilience, life we review.

Not merely a medical term,

But a lesson, from which we learn.

Riddle 128

A shadow of the past, yet present still,

A test of society's will.

Not just a cough, but deeper woes,

In every breath, the challenge grows.

A battle not of one, but all,

In prevention, we heed the call.

A journey through time, through care,

In every story, a shared affair.

Not just an illness of the lung,

But a reminder, of songs unsung.

Not merely a disease to cure,

But a fight, ongoing and pure.

Riddle 129

A fog that descends, erasing tales,

Where memory's ship, no longer sails.

Not just a loss, but a fading light,

In the darkness, seeking sight.

A challenge of identity, of known,

In every moment, seeds are sown.

A journey through the mist, hand in hand,

With love and patience, we stand.

Not just a condition, but a fading away,

In every goodbye, a wish to stay.

Not merely a medical term's claim,

But a quest for dignity, all the same.

Riddle 130

A shadow on health, a fear unspoken,

In every diagnosis, lives are broken.

Not just a tumor, but a battle fierce,

In every treatment, hope we pierce.

A challenge of body, spirit, mind,

In community, strength we find.

A journey of courage, of tears, of fight,

In darkness, seeking light.

Not just an illness, but a rallying cry,

In every moment, a reason why.

Not merely a disease's toll,

But a testament to the resilient soul.

Riddle 131

A shadow lurking in depths unseen,

Where wellness ends and fears convene.

In hidden folds, it makes its bed,

A silent threat, a growing dread.

Not just a condition of the gut,

But a battle, no ifs or but,

Screening's call, a chance to fight,

In early catch, lies the light.

A challenge deep within, so stark,

Prompting journeys from the dark.

Not merely an illness's name,

But a quest for health, to reclaim.

Riddle 132

A sweet betrayal, a body's plight,

Where sugar turns from friend to blight.

In veins it flows, too rich, too rife,

Altering the essence of life.

A daily dance of numbers and food,

In balance, a life's mood.

Not just a tale of insulin's grace,

But a journey, a lifelong race.

A condition shared by young and old,

In its grasp, life's stories told.

Not merely a disease of part,

But a challenge of the heart.

Riddle 133

A virus hidden, a whisper of fate,

Challenging life, love, and hate.

In silence it moves, in shadows it binds,

Seeking solace, it rarely finds.

A battle not just of body, but soul,

In unity, a collective goal.

Not just a sickness, but a societal test,

In compassion, we find our best.

A journey through stigma, through fear,

With hope and care drawn near.

Not merely an illness's strain,

But a world's pain, to contain.

Riddle 134

A miner's plight within the vein,

Where crystals form and cause pain.

Tiny stones with mighty might,

Turning days to sleepless night.

A journey through the body's tract,

In their wake, the impact.

Not just a condition of diet's fault,

But a challenge, a bodily assault.

A tale of water's power missed,

In prevention, lies the twist.

Not merely an ailment to bemoan,

But a call to wellness, to be known.

Riddle 135

A bite so small, a danger vast,

In nature's beauty, shadows cast.

A tick's gift, unwelcome, true,

Changing life's hues and cue.

In joints and hearts, it makes its mark,

From light into the dark.

Not just a tale of outdoor spree,

But a caution, a plea.

A challenge met with early test,

In treatment, lies the quest.

Not merely an infection's claim,

But a reminder of nature's game.

Riddle 136

A fever's rise, a chill's descent,

On tiny wings, the threat is sent.

In blood it swims, a parasite's dream,

Turning health into a scream.

A battle fought with net and pill,

In prevention, lies the will.

Not just a sickness of the tropic's kiss,

But a global fight, hit or miss.

A condition shared by land and air,

In its history, a collective care.

Not merely a disease to treat,

But a foe to finally defeat.

Riddle 137

A modern plight of excess and want,

Where calories haunt and taunt.

In every bite, a story told,

Of health bought, sold, and scrolled.

A challenge not of weight alone,

But of lifestyle, tone, and bone.

Not just a condition seen by eye,

But a deeper question of how and why.

A societal mirror, reflecting back,

In nutrition's lack, the track.

Not merely a personal fight,

But a shared plight, in light.

Riddle 138

A mind's maze, complex, profound,

Where reality and dreams are bound.

Voices whisper, unseen seen,

In between, life's screen.

A challenge of perception's core,

In understanding, so much more.

Not just a tale of medicine's quest,

But of humanity, at its best.

A journey through stigma, through fear,

With empathy drawn near.

Not merely a diagnosis to label,

But a life, a story, able.

Riddle 139

A tale of blood, reshaped, remiss,

In every cell, a crisis.

A genetic whisper, passed down,

In every smile, a hidden frown.

A battle not just of the body's make,

But of resilience, daybreak.

Not just a condition of the blood's flow,

But a story of life, grow.

A challenge met with courage, might,

In knowledge, research, light.

Not merely an illness's path,

But a journey, a math.

Riddle 140

A craft of healing, layer by layer,

In burns and wounds, a prayer.

A tale of renewal, skin anew,

In art and science, cue.

Not just a procedure of cut and place,

But of hope, in space.

A challenge of body's canvas, broad,

In recovery's road, trod.

Not merely a medical act,

But a life, intact.

In grafting's skill, a new dawn,

In healing's song, drawn.

Riddle 141

In the quiet of night, a silence breaks,

With a gasp, a snore, in fits and shakes.

Not just a pause in night's sweet song,

But a signal something's wrong.

A battle unseen, in the dark, they fight,

For every breath, with all their might.

Not merely snoring, but a deeper tale,

Where breath is caught, then fails.

A mask, a machine, may come to aid,

Ensuring rest, no longer delayed.

Not just a nuisance, but a serious call,

For health's sake, a concern for all.

Riddle 142

A butterfly gland, so small, so keen,

In its balance, health is seen.

Too slow, too fast, it can sway,

Affecting nights and days.

Not just energy, weight, or mood,

But a whole system's interlude.

A pill, a test, often the fix,

In its rhythm, life's mix.

Not merely a whisper in the throat,

But a note, on which lifeboats float.

A silent keeper of metabolic tales,

In its balance, health scales.

Riddle 143

Twisted paths, where blood should flow,

But instead, they bulge, and show.

Not just a cosmetic fret or sigh,

But a sign, circulation's awry.

Legs tired, heavy, bearing the mark,

Of veins that have lost their spark.

Not merely lines of age or fate,

But a sign, to investigate.

Compression, elevation, sometimes a zap,

To ease the journey on the map.

Not just an ailment of the vain,

But a circulatory refrain.

Riddle 144

A leap across species, unseen,

Where once was barrier, now not keen.

Not just a story of animal to man,

But a warning, to understand.

A virus, bacteria, parasite's ride,

From wild or companion, side by side.

Not merely a tale of nature's call,

But a reminder, we're part of it all.

Prevention, care, a global plea,

To live in harmony, respectfully.

Not just diseases that roam or fly,

But a shared fate, under one sky.

Riddle 145

With needles fine, a map is drawn,

On skin's canvas, from dusk till dawn.

Not just a prick, or a simple poke,

But a flow of energy, to invoke.

Ancient wisdom, modern embrace,

In every point, health's trace.

Not merely an alternative plea,

But a practice, deep and free.

Pain, stress, and so much more,

In its method, an open door.

Not just tradition, but a healing art,

In body's map, plays its part.

Riddle 146

A transformation, not just of size,

But of life, before one's eyes.

Not merely a reduction, a cut, or a trim,

But a journey, from within.

A choice, for health, for life, for self,

A commitment, to wellness, to wealth.

Not just a surgical act, but a start,

Of a journey, taken by heart.

Weight's burden, lifted with care,

In its wake, a new life to wear.

Not merely about what's lost, but found,

In health's embrace, profound.

Riddle 147

A battle waged within, a toxic fray,

Where cells both good and bad may pay.

Not just a treatment, but a siege,

Against cancer, a relentless league.

Hair may fall, and strength may wane,

But hope, in heart, remains.

Not merely poison, but a potion rare,

In life's balance, a careful snare.

A journey through the toughest storm,

With healing, as its norm.

Not just a trial of body, but soul,

In its quest, a hopeful goal.

Riddle 148

A boost, a shield, a warrior's aid,

In body's own defense, not to fade.

Not just a treatment, but a fight,

With one's own cells, in cancer's night.

Harnessing power, innate, profound,

Where hope and healing abound.

Not merely a drug, but a key,

Unlocking immunity's spree.

A battle not fought alone, but together,

In body's cause, a tether.

Not just a path, but a revolution,

In cancer's fight, a contribution.

Riddle 149

Invisible beams, a targeted might,

Against tumors hidden from sight.

Not just a ray, but a precise art,

In cancer's cure, plays its part.

A balance of harm, and heal, so fine,

Where science and hope align.

Not merely destruction, but a careful dance,

In every dose, a chance.

A fight not just of flesh, but fate,

In every session, hope we create.

Not just a burden, but a beam of light,

In darkness, offering fight.

Riddle 150

With arms of steel, a surgeon's aid,

Precision and skill, in metal laid.

Not just a machine, but a guiding hand,

In surgery's land, it stands.

A future of healing, less pain, more gain,

Where scars are small, recovery's gain.

Not merely a tool, but a revolution,

In surgical evolution.

A dance of tech, flesh, and bone,

In its grace, progress is shown.

Not just an operation, but an art,

In healing's future, plays its part.

Riddle 151

A gift of life, from one to another,

A gesture profound, like no other.

Not just an organ, but a chance anew,

For hearts to beat, and lungs to breathe true.

A journey of hope, through science and care,

In matching and timing, nothing to spare.

Not merely a procedure, but a bond,

Where life and love go beyond.

A tale of survival, of generosity vast,

In this act, life's shadows are cast.

Not just a surgery, but a miracle's play,

In transplantation, hope's ray.

Riddle 152

A machine that breathes, when you cannot,

A lifeline, in battles fought.

Not just a device, but a whisper of air,

Giving moments, precious and rare.

In ICU's silence, it hums and it sings,

Of life, and the hope it brings.

Not merely equipment, but a bridge to mend,

In critical times, a vital friend.

A guardian of breath, of life's delicate flame,

In its rhythm, a name.

Not just a support, but a crucial fight,

In darkness, it offers light.

Riddle 153

A comfort in times, when cure is no more,

A solace, when life's at its core.

Not just medicine, but a touch, a word,

In this care, heartbeats are heard.

A journey together, patient and kin,

In compassion, we all win.

Not merely a treatment, but a way to be,

In life's final chapter, a sea.

A practice of kindness, of dignity, grace,

In its embrace, a sacred space.

Not just an end, but a quality found,

In palliative care, love is profound.

Riddle 154

A peek inside, with a lens so small,

Exploring joints, without a large incall.

Not just a look, but a fix, a mend,

In tiny incisions, healing's trend.

A knee, a shoulder, places tight,

Where pain once lurked, now light.

Not merely surgery, but a scope, a view,

In recovery, life anew.

A technique of precision, of minimal mark,

In its path, a spark.

Not just a procedure, but a way to heal,

In arthroscopy, movement's zeal.

Riddle 155

A field of thought, where right meets care,

In decisions tough, and choices rare.

Not just a study, but a moral guide,

In ethics, where values reside.

A balance of benefit, risk, and right,

In healthcare's day and night.

Not merely philosophy, but action's core,

In treatment, research, and more.

A compass in science, in life's delicate dance,

In its questions, a chance.

Not just a theory, but practice real,

In biomedical ethics, humanity's seal.

Riddle 156

A sudden halt, in life's rhythm and beat,

Where heart and breath no longer meet.

Not just a pause, but an urgent call,

For help, for action, before the fall.

A moment of crisis, of survival's test,

In quick response, hope's best.

Not merely a condition, but a race against time,

In every second, a climb.

A challenge of life, of fate's hand,

In its wake, a stand.

Not just a medical term, but a plea,

In cardiac arrest, life's key.

Riddle 157

A dialogue of change, of thought, and mind,

Where patterns broken, new paths we find.

Not just a talk, but a strategy, a plan,

In mental health, a fan.

A tool for coping, for growth, for life,

Cutting through distress, like a knife.

Not merely therapy, but a skill, a way,

In thoughts and actions, day by day.

A practice of mindfulness, of reflection, care,

In CBT, a stair.

Not just an intervention, but a journey shared,

In mental health, prepared.

Riddle 158

A heart overwhelmed, a struggle to pump,

In fluid's embrace, a lump.

Not just a failure, but a fight to breathe,

In every beat, a sheathe.

A condition of wear, of time, of life,

In symptoms, strife.

Not merely a diagnosis, but a call,

For care, for change, for all.

A battle of balance, of fluid, and heart,

In treatment, a start.

Not just an ailment, but a life's review,

In congestive heart failure, a clue.

Riddle 159

A path narrowed, where blood should flow,

In arteries' journey, a slow.

Not just a block, but a risk, a sign,

Of hearts in trouble, in line.

A challenge of lifestyle, of genetics, too,

In prevention, a clue.

Not merely a condition, but a wake-up call,

In health's maintenance, not to fall.

A tale of vessels, of life's essence,

In care, a presence.

Not just a disease, but a pathway's test,

In coronary care, a quest.

Riddle 160

A chill so deep, it heals, it mends,

In cold's embrace, pain ends.

Not just a freeze, but a therapeutic touch,

In its grip, much.

A treatment cold, yet warmly met,

In recovery's net.

Not merely ice, but science, art,

In body's heal, a part.

A therapy of extreme, of contrast, bright,

In cold, a light.

Not just a method, but a path, a way,

In cryotherapy, play.

Riddle 161

A canvas worn, now seeks to mend,

With a tool that smooths, it tends to blend.

Not just a scrub, but deeper still,

It's art and skill, against the will

Of scars and time, to make anew,

A visage bright, and texture true.

A gentle sand, a careful graze,

In its path, beauty's maze.

Not merely cosmetic, but a renewal deep,

Where skin's stories, in confidence, keep.

A transformation, not just of skin,

But of how we feel, deep within.

Riddle 162

A machine's embrace, to cleanse, to clear,

When kidneys falter, this gear appears.

A cycle of life, through plastic veins,

It takes, it gives, it sustains.

Not just a process, but a lease anew,

On life, on moments, on morning's dew.

A bridge of time, till healing's hand,

Or a transplant, in life's sand.

Not merely treatment, but a passage, a tide,

Where hope and life, in balance, reside.

A ritual of cleansing, rhythmically bound,

In its hum, life's pulse is found.

Riddle 163

A map of thought, of dream, of mind,

In squiggles and lines, stories find.

Not just a test, but a journey deep,

Into consciousness, a leap.

A symphony of neurons, in electric dance,

In patterns, a chance.

To diagnose, to understand,

In waves, a brain's land.

Not merely data, but a window clear,

Into the soul, far and near.

A testament to the unseen,

In its lines, thought's sheen.

Riddle 164

A mystery deep, of pain and fog,

A battle daily, a tireless slog.

Not just an ache, but a storm widespread,

In muscles and mind, a thread.

A quest for relief, for solace, for peace,

In therapies' embrace, a lease.

Not merely symptoms, but a life's rearrange,

In pursuit of comfort, a range.

A challenge of being, of feeling, of thought,

In its grasp, lives are wrought.

Not just an ailment, but a journey profound,

In its whisper, life's sound.

Riddle 165

A path rerouted, a journey new,

Where food's voyage, is bid adieu.

Not just a surgery, but a change of life,

In habits, in health, a strife.

A decision bold, a commitment strong,

In a body's chorus, a new song.

Not merely a procedure, but a turn,

Where from past ways, we learn.

A gateway to a future bright,

In weight's challenge, a light.

Not just a loss, but a gain,

In life's quality, a new lane.

Riddle 166

A silent storm, in liver's hold,

A tale of inflammation, old.

Not just a virus, but a thief of health,

In stealth, it moves, in stealth.

A battle of immunity, a fight to win,

Against a foe, unseen, within.

Not merely an illness, but a quest,

For cure, for care, for rest.

A spectrum wide, of A to C,

In its grasp, a plea.

Not just a condition, but a warning,

In health's morning, a dawning.

Riddle 167

A body's rebellion, subtle, sure,

Where sugar's key, fits no more.

Not just a term, but a life's twist,

In health's fabric, a persist.

A challenge daily, of diet, of pill,

In balance's quest, a skill.

Not merely a syndrome, but a sign,

Of times, of lifestyle, in line.

A precursor, a shadow, a threat,

In its wake, a net.

Not just a resistance, but a call,

To heed, to act, to forestall.

Riddle 168

A yellow tale, in eye and skin,

Where liver's struggle, seen within.

Not just a hue, but a sign,

Of bile's dance, out of line.

A newborn's challenge, an adult's fear,

In its color, caution's near.

Not merely a symptom, but a clue,

Of health's puzzle, through and through.

A warning light, on body's dash,

In health's journey, a flash.

Not just a color, but a tale,

In diagnosis, we unveil.

Riddle 169

A dairy's dilemma, in gut's protest,

Where milk's delight, fails the test.

Not just a discomfort, but a sign,

Of enzymes' absence, in line.

A battle of bloating, of distress,

In diet's adjust, a guess.

Not merely an allergy, but a lack,

In digestion's track, a crack.

A choice of alternatives, a lifestyle's bend,

In nutrition's journey, a blend.

Not just intolerance, but a shift,

In dietary gifts, a lift.

Riddle 170

A choice, a chance, in health's fight,

Where breast's loss, brings a light.

Not just a surgery, but a stand,

Against a threat, hand in hand.

A journey of courage, of fear, of hope,

On recovery's slope, a rope.

Not merely a loss, but a gain,

In survival's name, a chain.

A testament to strength, to life,

In cancer's battle, a knife.

Not just an operation, but a path,

In healing's aftermath, a bath.

Riddle 171

A slender tube's journey, not taken by choice,

From nostril to stomach, it finds its voice.

A lifeline for nutrition, a passage so clear,

For those who cannot eat, it draws near.

Not just a simple tube, but a route of care,

In healing's journey, it takes its share.

A bridge between the need and the feed,

In its placement, hope's seed.

Not merely a method, but a silent plea,

For recovery's chance, a key.

A whisper of life, in plastic's guise,

In its length, wellness lies.

Riddle 172

A tale of wear, of joints in despair,

Where movement's grace becomes rare.

Not just an ache, but a gradual theft,

Of ease and fluidity, left bereft.

A story told in every bend, twist, and turn,

In its grasp, for relief, we yearn.

Not merely aging's expected guest,

But a challenge, a daily test.

A dance slowed down by time's own hand,

In its rhythm, we understand.

Not just a condition, but life's wear and tear,

In every step, a silent prayer.

Riddle 173

A fury within, a fire so keen,

Where digestion's peace is rarely seen.

Not just a discomfort, but a true battle's rage,

In its storm, the body's cage.

A gland inflamed, in revolt so dire,

In every pang, a warning fire.

Not merely an illness, but a wake-up call,

For care, for vigilance, above all.

A testament to life's fragile chain,

In its healing, a regain.

Not just an ailment, but a journey through,

In its path, resilience anew.

Riddle 174

A life transformed, in a moment's twist,

Where movement's bounty is truly missed.

Not just a condition, but a new way to see,

The world, the self, in a different key.

A challenge of body, but not of mind,

In its test, strength we find.

Not merely a diagnosis, but a life's course,

In its waters, a different force.

A story of courage, of spirit, of heart,

In life's canvas, a new start.

Not just a limitation, but a boundless sea,

In its depths, a discovery to be.

Riddle 175

A sculptor's touch, on the bridge so central,

Transforming, refining, with intent so gentle.

Not just a surgery, but an art so fine,

Where form and function beautifully align.

A quest for balance, for breath, for grace,

In every line, a perfect trace.

Not merely cosmetic, but a deeper quest,

For confidence, for breathing, at its best.

A change so subtle, yet profound,

In its outcome, harmony found.

Not just an operation, but a transformation,

In its detail, a new foundation.

Riddle 176

A curve, a bend, not chosen, found,

Where straight lines are rarely bound.

Not just a posture, but a deeper strain,

In its arc, a silent pain.

A journey of adjustments, of care, of might,

In its challenge, a fight.

Not merely a condition, but a path to walk,

In every therapy, in every talk.

A testament to resilience, to strength within,

In its curve, a win.

Not just a diagnosis, but a life's embrace,

In its course, a grace.

Riddle 177

A ring, a buzz, in solitude's hall,

Where silence should be, it takes its toll.

Not just a sound, but an unseen guest,

In its presence, a quest.

A challenge of perception, of peace, of mind,

In its whisper, a bind.

Not merely a symptom, but a deeper cry,

For understanding, for relief, to try.

A constant companion, unwelcome, true,

In its melody, a clue.

Not just an ailment, but a journey's sound,

In its path, wisdom found.

Riddle 178

A storm within, a rebellion raw,

Where comfort's law is no more.

Not just discomfort, but a true battle's field,

In its fury, hidden shield.

A quest for calm, for healing's touch,

In every flare, a clutch.

Not merely an illness, but a life's storm,

In its weather, a form.

A testament to endurance, to hope's might,

In its darkness, a light.

Not just a condition, but a path to tread,

In its journey, a thread.

Riddle 179

A journey through rivers deep within,

Where life's essence takes its spin.

Not just an operation, but a path so clear,

In its course, a cheer.

A challenge of flow, of life, of breath,

In its success, a death.

Not merely a procedure, but a craft so keen,

In its stitches, unseen.

A testament to skill, to art, to care,

In its flow, a share.

Not just a surgery, but a life's renew,

In its passage, a view.

Riddle 180

A tale of healing, of time, of skin,

Where recovery's journey does begin.

Not just a bandage, but a tender touch,

In its gentleness, a clutch.

A challenge of patience, of nurture, of might,

In its darkness, a light.

Not merely treatment, but a compassionate art,

In its practice, a heart.

A testament to resilience, to life's force,

In its process, a course.

Not just a task, but a healing embrace,

In its pace, grace.

Riddle 181

From one kind to another, a gift does pass,

A leap across species, bold and vast.

Not just a transplant, but a bridge so rare,

In hope's pursuit, a daring affair.

A heart, a kidney, cells that bind,

Seeking compatibility, a match to find.

Not merely science, but a boundary crossed,

In life's web, intricately tossed.

A quest for solutions, in shortages stark,

Lighting survival's hopeful spark.

Not just medicine, but a fusion of life,

In its essence, a cut like a knife.

Riddle 182

A healing flow, of breath and pose,

Where calm and strength, gracefully compose.

Not just a practice, but a therapy deep,

In its embrace, wellness we reap.

A bend, a stretch, a mindful state,

In every movement, balance we create.

Not merely exercise, but a holistic art,

Healing body, mind, and heart.

A journey within, through quiet and storm,

In its passage, transformations form.

Not just a session, but a life's embrace,

In its rhythm, a healing grace.

Riddle 183

A journey begins, where life's sparked anew,

In tubes and whispers, a hopeful view.

Not just a transfer, but a precise dance,

In fertility's realm, a chance.

A fusion of science, of hope, of life,

Cutting through impossibility, like a knife.

Not merely a procedure, but a dream cast,

In its moment, futures vast.

A blend of nature and human craft,

Seeking to harness life's draft.

Not just a method, but a bridge to birth,

In its crossing, a new earth.

Riddle 184

A guardian against the clot's stealthy tread,

Ensuring blood's flow, not dread.

Not just a medicine, but a shield in vein,

In its presence, safety's gain.

A battle within, of fluidity and fight,

Keeping health in sight.

Not merely drugs, but lifesavers keen,

In their role, unseen.

A dance of chemistry and care,

In its balance, life's fare.

Not just a treatment, but a vital key,

In its use, freedom's spree.

Riddle 185

A renewal of essence, of blood's own source,

In illness's journey, a powerful force.

Not just a transplant, but a rebirth, profound,

In its success, life unbound.

A match of marrow, of genetics, a tie,

In its attempt, hope's high.

Not merely a procedure, but a gift of life,

Cutting through disease, like a knife.

A bridge to healing, to a future bright,

In its passage, a fight.

Not just medicine, but a miracle's thread,

In its weaving, dread is shed.

Riddle 186

A spiral journey, in beams and slice,

Revealing the hidden, at a price.

Not just a scan, but an explorer's gaze,

In its depth, mysteries amaze.

A circle of light, of X-ray's kiss,

Capturing images, miss nor dismiss.

Not merely a machine, but a vision deep,

In its findings, secrets we keep.

A window to the inner, to the core,

In its revelation, much more.

Not just a procedure, but a guide to heal,

In its clarity, truth we feel.

Riddle 187

A careful parting, layer by layer,

Seeking knowledge, a truth's player.

Not just a cutting, but an inquiry deep,

In its study, secrets we reap.

A journey through the silent, the still,

Understanding life's fill.

Not merely a task, but a learning keen,

In its process, unseen.

A dialogue with the silent, a respectful bond,

In its passage, answers found.

Not just a method, but a bridge to know,

In its reveal, wisdom's flow.

Riddle 188

Dancers in fluid, a balance so fine,

In their rhythm, health's line.

Not just particles, but life's charge they carry,

In their dance, merry and vary.

A harmony of sodium, potassium's play,

In their balance, life's sway.

Not merely elements, but a vital beat,

In their motion, life's treat.

A symphony in blood, in sweat, in tear,

In their presence, life's cheer.

Not just a science, but a life's essence,

In their measure, health's presence.

Riddle 189

A whisper of life, a heartbeat's song,

In its rhythm, strong and long.

Not just listening, but a guarding close,

In its beat, a life's propose.

A connection deep, a bond before birth,

In its sound, life's worth.

Not merely a procedure, but a celebration,

In its frequency, a foundation.

A vigil of care, of anticipation's hold,

In its story, futures told.

Not just a task, but a love's embrace,

In its pattern, life's trace.

Riddle 190

A pressure unseen, a sight's slow steal,

In its grasp, a reality unreal.

Not just a condition, but a silent thief,

In its progress, disbelief.

A challenge of vision, of light's dimming door,

In its wake, seeking more.

Not merely an ailment, but a fight to see,

In its journey, a plea.

A testament to vigilance, to care's keen eye,

In its challenge, a sky.

Not just a diagnosis, but a life's adjust,

In its presence, trust.

Riddle 191

A healing approach, both wide and deep,

Where mind, body, spirit, in care we keep.

Not just one part, but the whole we see,

In nature's embrace, health's key.

A blend of traditions, new and old,

In its wisdom, stories told.

Not merely treatment, but balance and grace,

In wellness's journey, a gentle pace.

A symphony of healing, in harmony found,

In its practice, life's profound.

Not just a method, but a way to live,

In holistic care, love we give.

Riddle 192

A lifeline in tubes, a liquid's flow,

Direct to veins, where healing's aglow.

Not just a drip, but a vital stream,

Carrying hope, in every gleam.

A bridge to wellness, in fluids clear,

In its path, recovery near.

Not merely a method, but a rapid course,

In healing's journey, a powerful force.

A cascade of care, in silent vein,

In its whisper, health's regain.

Not just treatment, but life's essence,

In IV therapy, a presence.

Riddle 193

A marvel of engineering, in body's frame,

Where worn parts renewed, reclaim.

Not just a procedure, but a rebirth of sorts,

In mobility's dance, in sports.

A new lease on life, in metal and might,

Where every movement's a delight.

Not merely surgery, but transformation,

In movement's ease, a celebration.

A testament to science, to art, to care,

In its craft, life we dare.

Not just a fix, but a journey's restart,

In joint replacement, a heart.

Riddle 194

A shift in fuel, from sugar to fat,

Where weight loss and energy are at.

Not just a diet, but a change profound,

In its regime, health's sound.

A battle against carbs, a quest for lean,

In its practice, change is seen.

Not merely eating, but a lifestyle's art,

In ketogenic ways, a smart start.

A path to wellness, in fats embrace,

In its journey, a new pace.

Not just a fad, but a science's claim,

In ketogenic diet, a flame.

Riddle 195

A needle's journey, in spine's embrace,

To draw the fluid, in careful grace.

Not just a test, but a window clear,

To what's within, to what's dear.

A clue to maladies, hidden deep,

In its draw, secrets we keep.

Not merely a procedure, but insight's door,

In diagnosis, a core.

A moment of discomfort, for knowledge's gain,

In lumbar puncture, a lane.

Not just a puncture, but a guide,

In spinal mysteries, we confide.

Riddle 196

A guardian of beginnings, of life so new,

Where tiny breaths, and strength accrue.

Not just a field, but a tender fight,

In neonates, a light bright.

A care for the smallest, in their first quest,

In its arms, life's test.

Not merely medicine, but love's pure form,

In neonatology, a storm.

A journey of care, from first breaths drawn,

In its practice, dawn's yawn.

Not just a specialty, but a heart's call,

In neonatology, love's thrall.

Riddle 197

A relief in pain, in doses small,

Where relief and risk, in shadow's pall.

Not just a medicine, but a double-edged sword,

In its use, caution's word.

A balm for suffering, but a chain for some,

In its grip, wills numb.

Not merely drugs, but a debate's core,

In opioids, a lore.

A quest for balance, in pain's relief,

In its story, joy and grief.

Not just a prescription, but a societal tide,

In opioids, a divide.

Riddle 198

A mother's challenge, hidden within,

Where birth's journey, delicate, thin.

Not just a condition, but a careful wait,

In its outcome, fate.

A story of life, in suspense held,

In its course, hearts swelled.

Not merely an obstacle, but a path to tread,

In pregnancy's book, a thread.

A whisper of caution, in birth's song,

In placenta previa, where hopes belong.

Not just a term, but a journey's part,

In maternal love, a heart.

Riddle 199

A battle of wills, in smoke's embrace,

Where habit and health, face to face.

Not just a choice, but a war to win,

In quitting's quest, begin.

A myriad of aids, in fight's array,

In therapies, hope's ray.

Not merely a stop, but a life reclaimed,

In smoke-free breaths, named.

A journey from addiction's shadow,

In therapies, a meadow.

Not just cessation, but a brighter day,

In quitting smoking, a way.

Riddle 200

A thief of sight, in vessels' weave,

Where light and dark, deceive.

Not just a disease, but a silent creep,

In vision's depth, a leap.

A challenge to sight, in blur and blind,

In its grasp, binds.

Not merely damage, but a call to care,

In eyes' health, a share.

A story of vision, slowly told,

In retinopathy, bold.

Not just an ailment, but a sight's plea,

In vision's care, a key.

Riddle 201

A silent storm that brews within,

A battle fierce, beneath the skin.

Not just an infection, but a cascade wild,

Where defenses falter, in turmoil piled.

A race against time, in vessels deep,

Where shadows of mortality creep.

Not merely sickness, but a systemic fight,

In its grip, day turns to night.

A challenge of survival, stark and real,

In its presence, life's zeal.

Not just a condition, but an urgent plea,

For intervention, swift and free.

Riddle 202

A passage forged, when breath's at stake,

A vital route, we undertake.

Not just a procedure, but a lifeline made,

In its channel, fears fade.

A window to the wind, for air so sweet,

Where lungs and life, in breath, meet.

Not merely an opening, but a bridge to breathe,

In its presence, relief we weave.

A testament to resilience, to life's demand,

In its making, hope's hand.

Not just an act of medical art,

But a journey's crucial part.

Riddle 203

A burning tale, a discomfort deep,

Where bacteria in shadows creep.

Not just a nuisance, but a fiery quest,

In its wake, no rest.

A battle in the waterways, unseen,

Where pain and urgency convene.

Not merely a symptom, but a sign to heed,

In its message, caution's seed.

A common plight, yet hidden so,

In its grip, discomforts grow.

Not just an ailment, but a call to care,

In its treatment, relief we share.

Riddle 204

A hidden threat, a bulge unseen,

In vessel's wall, it lies between.

Not just a swelling, but a silent dare,

In its presence, a scare.

A ticking time, within life's stream,

Where rupture's risk, is not just a dream.

Not merely a bubble, but a looming fight,

In its shadow, a fright.

A challenge of life, of fate's own hand,

In its risk, a stand.

Not just a condition, but a whispered call,

For vigilance, above all.

Riddle 205

A gift of life, in red's own flow,

From one to another, in hope, it goes.

Not just a transfer, but a shared embrace,

In its journey, a trace.

A bond of survival, in tubes entwined,

Where life's essence, is refined.

Not merely a procedure, but a saving grace,

In its gift, life's race.

A testament to generosity's might,

In its offering, light.

Not just a treatment, but a connection deep,

In its passage, hope we keep.

Riddle 206

A curtain lifted, from eye's own view,

Where blurred worlds, become anew.

Not just a removal, but a vision restored,

In its clarity, life adored.

A journey from shadow, to light's embrace,

Where sights and colors, find their place.

Not merely an operation, but a dawn bright,

In its success, delight.

A gift of sight, so clear, so bold,

In its making, stories told.

Not just a change of lens, but a life's gain,

In its procedure, a new domain.

Riddle 207

A silent peril, in depth's own hold,

Where blood's journey turns cold.

Not just a clot, but a lurking threat,

In its trap, a net.

A challenge of flow, of life's own course,

In its presence, a force.

Not merely a block, but a call to action,

In its risk, a fraction.

A tale of caution, of vigilance due,

In its lesson, a clue.

Not just an ailment, but a journey's bend,

In its care, a mend.

Riddle 208

A heart's whisper, in waves told,

A story of rhythm, of life, bold.

Not just an echo, but a vision deep,

In its sound, secrets keep.

A dance of chambers, in harmony's play,

Where life's pulse, finds its way.

Not merely a test, but a glimpse within,

In its rhythm, life's spin.

A testament to the beat's own song,

In its cadence, strong.

Not just a procedure, but a heartbeat's tale,

In its reveal, a sail.

Riddle 209

A tale of breaks, of healing's art,

Where bones and care, play their part.

Not just a mend, but a journey back,

In its path, no lack.

A challenge of patience, of time, of skill,

In recovery's will.

Not merely a fix, but a restoration,

In its care, a foundation.

A testament to resilience, to body's might,

In its healing, a light.

Not just a treatment, but a path to regain,

In its course, a refrain.

Riddle 210

A map of life, in codes told,

Where stories of genes, unfold.

Not just advice, but a guiding light,

In its wisdom, insight.

A journey through possibilities, risks, and dreams,

Where future's fabric, seams.

Not merely a session, but a deep dive,

In understanding, we thrive.

A testament to knowledge's power,

In its depth, a tower.

Not just a conversation, but a life's guide,

In its counsel, we confide.

Riddle 211

A gland in haste, too swift its pace,

In its rush, life's race.

Not just a flutter, but a storm within,

Where warmth and tremors begin.

A battle of speed, unseen, unfelt,

In its fervor, wellness melts.

Not merely a symptom, but a sign so clear,

In its whisper, we hear.

A tale of excess, of too much fire,

In its wake, a tire.

Not just an ailment, but a body's plea,

For balance, for harmony.

Riddle 212

A weight unseen, inside the skull,

Where thoughts and dreams, it tries to cull.

Not just a number, but a critical sign,

In its balance, a fine line.

A battle against the squeeze, the press,

In its grip, distress.

Not merely a condition, but a dire quest,

For relief, for rest.

A silent force, pushing within,

In its challenge, a din.

Not just a pressure, but a threat to quell,

In its story, much to tell.

Riddle 213

A youth's trial, sweet's betrayal,

Where insulin becomes the grail.

Not just a prickle, but a life's change,

In routines, rearrange.

A tale of vigilance, of care, of might,

In every meal, a fight.

Not merely a disease, but a journey's start,

In each drop, a heart.

A challenge of balance, of blood's own song,

In its rhythm, strong.

Not just a condition, but a test of spirit,

In its whisper, we hear it.

Riddle 214

A vision restored, in cornea's grace,

Where light and sight, embrace.

Not just a surgery, but a gift of view,

In colors, in hue.

A tale of clarity, of worlds anew,

In each blink, a review.

Not merely a procedure, but a leap,

In its promise, a peep.

A craft of precision, of delicate hand,

In its touch, a land.

Not just an operation, but sight's reprise,

In its success, skies.

Riddle 215

A flow restrained, in tissues' swell,

Where fluids linger, dwell.

Not just a swelling, but a journey slowed,

In its path, a load.

A tale of channels, blocked and tight,

In its presence, a fight.

Not merely a symptom, but a body's cry,

For movement, for a sigh.

A challenge of passage, of flow's own might,

In its course, light.

Not just a condition, but a quest for ease,

In its answer, release.

Riddle 216

A heart's alarm, in muscle's strain,

Where blood's flow wanes.

Not just a moment, but a life's pause,

In its beat, a cause.

A tale of blockage, of paths untrod,

In its wake, a nod.

Not merely an event, but a call to mend,

For habits, to bend.

A battle for survival, for breath, for life,

In its story, strife.

Not just an attack, but a change's birth,

In its lesson, worth.

Riddle 217

A cradle of hope, where smallest fight,

In warmth and care, day and night.

Not just a room, but a bridge of life,

In its walls, less strife.

A tale of beginnings, tender, frail,

In each breath, a sail.

Not merely a place, but a haven's grace,

For life, a base.

A journey of growth, of strength's own quest,

In its care, a nest.

Not just a unit, but a story's start,

In its heart, art.

Riddle 218

A bone's rebirth, in cut and heal,

Where structure's change, we deal.

Not just a slice, but a correction's aim,

In form and function, same.

A tale of alignment, of balance sought,

In its craft, thought.

Not merely a procedure, but a path to stride,

For comfort, a guide.

A challenge of precision, of surgeon's skill,

In its success, thrill.

Not just a surgery, but a life's amend,

In its outcome, a blend.

Riddle 219

A tale of nerves, distant and dim,

Where sensation's light, grows grim.

Not just a tingling, but a silent scream,

In its presence, a dream.

A journey of feeling, lost and found,

In its path, bound.

Not merely a condition, but a quest for cause,

In its mystery, a pause.

A challenge of movement, of touch's grace,

In its loss, a chase.

Not just an ailment, but a life's refrain,

In its story, pain.

Riddle 220

A beam precise, a scalpel's light,

Where cancer battles, take flight.

Not just a ray, but a focused fight,

In darkness, a sight.

A tale of healing, without a cut,

In its path, a shut.

Not merely a treatment, but a hope's lance,

In its aim, a chance.

A journey of cure, in gamma's glow,

In its reach, a bow.

Not just a surgery, but a silent grace,

In its touch, space.

Riddle 221

In the backbone's tale, where segments align,

A surgical craft, so fine.

Not just a joining, but a unity sought,

For pain and wear, battles fought.

A bridge of bone, metal, and graft,

In hopes that mobility is recast.

Not merely fixing, but restoring grace,

In each movement, a trace.

A testament to resolve, to mend,

In its outcome, a blend.

Not just a procedure, but a path to stand,

In fusion's craft, a hand.

Riddle 222

A whisper of warning, brief and stark,

Where blood's flow misses its mark.

Not just a shadow, but a prelude clear,

In its moment, fear.

A signal, fleeting, yet profound,

In its passage, bound.

Not merely a scare, but a call to heed,

In prevention, a lead.

A challenge to arteries, a cerebral fight,

In its recovery, light.

Not just an episode, but a beacon's flash,

In health's canvas, a dash.

Riddle 223

A window to the unseen, in waves it sings,

Where echoes shape, life's beginnings.

Not just a picture, but a revelation deep,

In its vision, secrets keep.

A pulse of sound, soft and profound,

In its frequency, bound.

Not merely viewing, but understanding's key,

In echoes, clarity.

A glimpse within, where life's script is penned,

In its display, a blend.

Not just imaging, but a bridge to see,

In ultrasound, discovery.

Riddle 224

A tale of joints, where fluid's restored,

In lubrication, movement adored.

Not just an injection, but a relief sought,

For stiffness and pain, battles fought.

A gel-like substance, in syringe borne,

In its arrival, hope reborn.

Not merely treating, but easing the glide,

In each step, a stride.

A therapy aimed at knees' embrace,

In its essence, a grace.

Not just a procedure, but a journey to ease,

In viscosupplementation, a peace.

Riddle 225

A quest for balance, in diet and scale,

Where discipline and guidance prevail.

Not just a plan, but a lifestyle's change,

In habits rearranged.

A journey of numbers, of meals, of sweat,

In its challenge, a bet.

Not merely losing, but gaining control,

In body and soul.

A commitment to health, to life, to self,

In its pursuit, wealth.

Not just a program, but a transformation's start,

In weight management, heart.

Riddle 226

A quest for moisture, in dryness' wake,

Where saliva's flow takes a break.

Not just a symptom, but a discomfort's tale,

In its remedy, we hail.

A battle against dryness, a quest for relief,

In treatments, belief.

Not merely managing, but restoring a sense,

In hydration, recompense.

A challenge of glands, of moisture's might,

In its care, a light.

Not just a condition, but a quality of life,

In xerostomia treatment, strife.

Riddle 227

A traveler's bane, in tropics spread,

Where mosquitoes dine, and fears are fed.

Not just a virus, but a fever's rage,

In history, a page.

A battle of immunity, a vaccine's grace,

In prevention, a race.

Not merely a disease, but a global fight,

In health's oversight.

A tale of jaundice, of aches, of pain,

In recovery, gain.

Not just an ailment, but a world's concern,

In yellow fever, learn.

Riddle 228

A pouch where food mistakenly strays,

In swallowing's maze, it stays.

Not just a pocket, but a hidden trap,

In dining, a gap.

A challenge of esophagus, a silent plight,

In its presence, a fight.

Not merely a condition, but a swallow's breach,

In treatment, reach.

A tale of discomfort, of meals not passed,

In its care, contrast.

Not just a diagnosis, but a lifestyle's tweak,

In Zenker's, relief we seek.

Riddle 229

Tools of aid, in life's daily grind,

Where ease and accessibility we find.

Not just gadgets, but freedom's keys,

In their use, ease.

A bridge over hurdles, large and small,

In their support, we stand tall.

Not merely accessories, but empowerment's form,

In independence, a norm.

A testament to innovation's quest,

In adaptive devices, life's zest.

Not just equipment, but a helping hand,

In their grace, we stand.

Riddle 230

A storm within, a membrane's plight,

Where bacteria invade, and defenses fight.

Not just an infection, but a critical race,

In its urgency, pace.

A battle of wills, of life, of breath,

In its grip, a test of death.

Not merely sickness, but a fight for the dawn,

In its wake, a new morn.

A tale of survival, of medicine's might,

In its challenge, a fight.

Not just a disease, but a wake-up call,

In bacterial meningitis, a wall.

Riddle 231

A shadow that grows, in the mind's quiet room,

Where laughter fades and fears loom.

Not just sadness, but a deeper shade,

Where light dims and hopes fade.

A battle unseen, fought day and night,

Seeking a flicker, a spark of light.

Not merely mood, but a storm within,

Where finding anchor is to begin.

A quest for solace, for some relief,

In understanding, lies belief.

Not just a condition, but a journey's start,

In healing the mind, the soul, the heart.

Riddle 232

A whisper of blood, in flow and in speed,

A sonic detective, to listen and heed.

Not just an echo, but a tale told in waves,

Of life coursing through invisible caves.

A dance of sound, high and low,

Revealing secrets, hidden below.

Not merely a test, but an exploration deep,

In its findings, trust we keep.

A melody of the body, in motion and rest,

In its rhythm, life's quest.

Not just a procedure, but a window to view,

In Doppler's song, life anew.

Riddle 233

A journey within, through passages tight,

Where mysteries unfold in artificial light.

Not just a voyage, but a quest to see,

What lies beneath, in mystery.

A camera's eye, on a flexible path,

Seeking answers, finding facts.

Not merely a look, but a discovery's chance,

In its vision, a glance.

A tale of the hidden, brought to day,

In its reveal, truth's way.

Not just an exploration, but a guide,

In endoscopy, secrets don't hide.

Riddle 234

A tale as old as time, yet fresh and bold,

Where one's waste becomes another's gold.

Not just a transfer, but a life's exchange,

In gut's flora, a range.

A battle of bacteria, good versus bad,

In its outcome, happy and sad.

Not merely a procedure, but a new lease on life,

In its essence, relief from strife.

A story of healing, of balance restored,

In its simplicity, health's accord.

Not just a treatment, but a revolution,

In FMT, a solution.

Riddle 235

A twilight's care, for the mind's gentle decline,

Where wisdom and sorrow, often entwine.

Not just a practice, but a tender art,

In aging's journey, a part.

A dialogue of memories, of joys and of fears,

In the evening of life, in the twilight of years.

Not merely a specialty, but a compassionate guide,

In geriatric hearts, hope resides.

A story of understanding, of patience and grace,

In its wisdom, a solace.

Not just a field, but a journey shared,

In geriatric care, hearts bared.

Riddle 236

A harbor of peace, as life's sun sets low,

Where comfort and dignity, gently flow.

Not just a place, but a philosophy of care,

In life's final chapter, a prayer.

A testament to love, to letting go,

In hospice's embrace, a soft glow.

Not merely an end, but a celebration of life,

In its passage, easing strife.

A journey of souls, in tender hands held,

In hospice care, hearts meld.

Not just a service, but a gentle goodbye,

In hospice's care, spirits fly.

Riddle 237

A fortress weakened, in the body's silent war,

Where defenses falter, and invaders score.

Not just a condition, but a life altered,

In its challenge, courage mustered.

A battle of immunity, in shadows fought,

Seeking safety, often sought.

Not merely a diagnosis, but a daily test,

In its journey, no rest.

A tale of resilience, of vulnerability,

In immunodeficiency, humanity.

Not just an ailment, but a quest to thrive,

In its struggle, spirits alive.

Riddle 238

A quest for relief, from swelling and pain,

Where needles and hope, often reign.

Not just a draw, but a search for cause,

In its procedure, a pause.

A tale of fluid, of secrets unveiled,

In its removal, comfort entailed.

Not merely a syringe's gentle pull,

But in aspiration, a lull.

A story of healing, of care so precise,

In its action, a device.

Not just a treatment, but a gesture of aid,

In joint aspiration, fears fade.

Riddle 239

A machine's embrace, a lifeline so pure,

Where blood finds a passage, a cure.

Not just a filter, but a second chance,

In its rhythm, a dance.

A battle against toxins, a cleansing deep,

In its vigil, health to keep.

Not merely a procedure, but a bridge to life,

In its hum, a strife.

A tale of survival, of endurance and will,

In dialysis, time stands still.

Not just a therapy, but a testament strong,

In kidney care, a song.

Riddle 240

A journey small, to the core so vital,

Where cells tell tales, in their recital.

Not just a sample, but a quest to know,

In its result, a show.

A tale of health, of concern, of care,

In its extract, a share.

Not merely a needle's quick descent,

But in biopsy, intent.

A story of discovery, of answers sought,

In its undertaking, thought.

Not just a procedure, but a path to heal,

In liver's tale, a zeal.

Riddle 241

In a world so small, where eyes can't see,

There's a dance of tools, in fine spree.

With precision and care, connections made,

Where healing's art is finely displayed.

Not just a stitch, but a weave so tight,

In tissues rejoined, a future bright.

A realm where detail and patience reign,

In each maneuver, hope's gain.

Not merely a procedure, but an art so fine,

In its craft, life's design.

A whisper of hope, in the tiniest space,

In microsurgery, a gentle grace.

Riddle 242

A tale of meals, where health's the aim,

In every bite, a different game.

Not just a diet, but a way to heal,

With every plate, a better feel.

A journey through foods, with wisdom shared,

In vitamins and minerals, care's prepared.

Not merely eating, but a thoughtful feast,

In its guidance, wellness increased.

A path of healing, with nature's best,

In nutritional therapy, a quest.

Not just a guide, but a lifestyle's embrace,

In every meal, health's trace.

Riddle 243

A journey of metal, wire, and band,

To straighten and align, as planned.

Not just a smile's cosmetic grace,

But a bite corrected, in its place.

A tale of patience, of years in wait,

For the perfect smile to create.

Not merely aesthetics, but a function's art,

In every adjustment, a new start.

A rite of passage, in youth's embrace,

In orthodontic braces, a trace.

Not just an ordeal, but a change profound,

In every smile, confidence found.

Riddle 244

A quest to quell, the body's cries,

In techniques and meds, relief lies.

Not just a symptom, but a challenge deep,

In its care, comfort we seek.

A journey through thresholds, high and low,

Finding solace, in pain's shadow.

Not merely treatment, but understanding's art,

In every strategy, a heart.

A battle against discomfort, a relentless fight,

In pain management, a light.

Not just a practice, but a compassionate plea,

In its embrace, pain flees.

Riddle 245

A measure of joy, of sorrow's weight,

In every question, fate.

Not just a survey, but a deeper dive,

In life's quality, we strive.

A tale of well-being, of days spent,

In its score, a life's content.

Not merely numbers, but stories told,

In each assessment, life's mold.

A reflection of living, in health's embrace,

In quality of life, a trace.

Not just an evaluation, but a guide to care,

In every answer, a share.

Riddle 246

A ghost of strep, in joints and heart,

Where inflammation's art.

Not just a fever, but a dance of pain,

In every symptom, a strain.

A tale of defense, misguided, lost,

In its aftermath, a cost.

Not merely an illness, but a warning clear,

In each prevention, a cheer.

A battle of past, in present's guise,

In rheumatic fever, a compromise.

Not just a disease, but a history's mark,

In every recovery, a spark.

Riddle 247

A journey of words, of sounds unbound,

Where expression's found.

Not just a lesson, but a bridge to speak,

In every voice, unique.

A tale of triumph, in trials small,

In every syllable, a call.

Not merely training, but a quest for voice,

In each session, a choice.

A path of communication, opened wide,

In speech therapy, a guide.

Not just a practice, but a life's embrace,

In every word, grace.

Riddle 248

A craft of life, in lab's design,

Where cells and scaffolds intertwine.

Not just a science, but creation's art,

In every tissue, a start.

A tale of regeneration, of form reborn,

In every structure, hope's sworn.

Not merely research, but a dream's pursuit,

In each project, life's root.

A journey of healing, from the very core,

In tissue engineering, a lore.

Not just an endeavor, but a future's key,

In every fiber, possibility.

Riddle 249

A treasure saved, from birth's first cry,

In cells so precious, hope lies high.

Not just a storage, but a legacy kept,

In every vial, a step adept.

A tale of potential, of futures bright,

In every deposit, a light.

Not merely a bank, but a safeguard, a chance,

In each collection, advance.

A promise of healing, in blood's embrace,

In umbilical care, grace.

Not just a choice, but a gift to behold,

In every cell, a story told.

Riddle 250

A quest for shields, against disease's night,

In every trial, a fight.

Not just a formula, but a hope's brew,

In every dose, life anew.

A tale of science, of patience, of might,

In every vial, light.

Not merely a process, but a global plea,

In each vaccine, a sea.

A journey of immunity, shared by all,

In vaccine's call, a wall.

Not just research, but a humanity's quest,

In every development, our best.

Riddle 251

In the realm where memory fades, a shadow plays,

Where yesterday's sun blurs in today's haze.

A tale of two halves, one lost, one confused,

In a dance of the mind, reality's muse.

Not born of age, but of a deficiency deep,

Where neurons starve, and protections sleep.

A phantom of forgetfulness, wandering halls,

Echoing in the brain's forsaken walls.

"Who are you?" it asks, with each passing hour,

Stealing the present, with an unseen power.

A riddle wrapped in mystery's embrace,

Seeking answers that time cannot erase.

Riddle 252

A secret whispered down the family tree,

Hidden in the code, for generations to see.

A legacy carried on wings so slight,

Borne by mothers, in sons it alights.

A puzzle locked within the X's embrace,

Challenging norms, a genetic chase.

Not just a disorder, but a marker's trail,

In its path, tales of hope and travail.

Where strength and vulnerability intertwine,

In the dance of chromosomes, a design.

A riddle of inheritance, so keen,

In its reveal, life's unseen screen.

Answers

1. Doctor
2. Nurse
3. Hospital
4. Clinic
5. Pharmacy
6. Ambulance
7. Triage Room
8. Medicine
9. Bills
10. Syrup
11. Stethoscope
12. Injection
13. Blood Pressure
14. Medical Record
15. Patient ID
16. ICU (Intensive Care Unit)
17. Emergency Unit
18. First Aid Kit
19. Health Insurance
20. Vaccination
21. Bandage
22. Thermometer
23. Physical Exam
24. Prescription
25. Wheelchair
26. Waiting Room
27. Appointment
28. Surgery
29. Recovery Room
30. Lab Test

31. X-Ray
32. MRI Scan
33. Ultrasound
34. Physical Therapy
35. Dental Care
36. Eye Examination
37. Check-up
38. Health Check
39. Flu Shot
40. Nutritionist
41. Pediatrician
42. Gynecologist
43. Orthopedist
44. Psychiatrist
45. Home Care
46. Nursing Home
47. Vitamins
48. Disinfectant
49. Health App
50. Cold Pack
51. Allergy Test
52. Blood Donation
53. Hearing Aid
54. Sunscreen
55. Antiseptic
56. Cough Drops
57. Health Fair
58. Oxygen Mask
59. Fitness Tracker
60. Medical Alert Bracelet
61. Anatomy
62. Physiology

95. Cholesterol
96. Diabetes
97. ECG (Electrocardiogram)
98. MRI (Magnetic Resonance Imaging)
99. Antibiotics
100. Epidemic
101. Pandemic
102. Biomedical Engineering
103. Health Informatics
104. Telemedicine
105. Clinical Trials
106. Stem Cells
107. Gene Therapy
108. Laparoscopy
109. Prosthetics
110. Vaccines
111. Anemia
112. Asthma
113. Autism
114. Bipolar Disorder
115. Cerebral Palsy
116. Dementia
117. Depression
118. Epilepsy
119. Heart Attack
120. Hypertension
121. Infertility
122. Leukemia
123. Melanoma
124. Meningitis
125. Osteoporosis
126. Parkinson's Disease

159.	Coronary Artery Disease
160.	Cryotherapy
161.	Dermabrasion
162.	Dialysis
163.	Electroencephalogram (EEG)
164.	Fibromyalgia
165.	Gastric Bypass
166.	Hepatitis
167.	Insulin Resistance
168.	Jaundice
169.	Lactose Intolerance
170.	Mastectomy
171.	Nasogastric Intubation
172.	Osteoarthritis
173.	Pancreatitis
174.	Quadriplegia
175.	Rhinoplasty
176.	Scoliosis
177.	Tinnitus
178.	Ulcerative Colitis
179.	Vascular Surgery
180.	Wound Care
181.	Xenotransplantation
182.	Yoga Therapy
183.	Zygote Intrafallopian Transfer (ZIFT)
184.	Anticoagulants
185.	Bone Marrow Transplant
186.	Computed Tomography (CT) Scan
187.	Dissection
188.	Electrolytes
189.	Fetal Monitoring
190.	Glaucoma

Don't miss out!

Visit the website below and you can sign up to receive emails whenever Said Al Azri publishes a new book. There's no charge and no obligation.

https://books2read.com/r/B-A-KSLCB-VEJVC

BOOKS 2 READ

Connecting independent readers to independent writers.

Also by Said Al Azri

Classics Reimagined: A Comedic Twist
Echoes of Venice: A Modern Tale of Redemption
Moby-Dick Reversed: A Whale's Humorous Account
Treasure Island: The Parrot's Perspective
Tom Sawyer: The Great Exaggerator

Family and Parenting Dynamics
From My Heart to Yours: Messages of Love and Learning for My
Child
Balancing Family Life: Strategies for Modern Parenting

Heartstrings: Tales of Valentine's Verse
Verses of the Heart: A Poetic Journey Through Love's Whimsy
Verses of the Heart 2: A Poetic Journey Through Love's Whimsy

Life, Hobbies, and Careers Series
From Amateur to Applause: A Beginner's Guide to Stand-Up Comedy

Living Fully After 50 Series
Rediscovering Hobbies and Passions After 50
Rediscovering Hobbies and Passions After 50, Book 2
Happiness in the Second Half: Finding Joy and Fulfillment After 50

Riddle Me This: A Professional Exploration in Poetry
The Techie's Riddles: IT-Inspired Poems for Curious Minds
The Healer's Verses: Medical Mysteries in Rhyme for the Analytical
Mind

www.ingramcontent.com/pod-product-compliance
Lightning Source LLC
Chambersburg PA
CBHW061427150726
47987CB00001B/120